'You may share my experience of pleasure when I survive a difficult consultation without harming the patient or of dealing with my lack of satisfaction without being punitive to client or staff. If so you will find this book illuminating, rewarding and instructive to read'. From the Foreword by Professor Paul Freeling, O.B.E.

When patient meets doctor, as well as engaging in a transaction with a clinical purpose, they react to one another as people. Their personalities and ability to make relationships in general also affect the professional interaction. As with other relationships, things can go wrong. The outcome of a consultation may not then be what was hoped for or intended on either side. What may be lost or not even achieved is a sense of working together with one another – hence the 'problem patient' or 'quack doctor'.

This book describes the factors that may complicate the clinical transaction between patient and doctor, emphasising and explaining the influence of often unconscious personal aspects. This is encompassed within a readily applied and concise model, which yields a fresh analysis and understanding. The insight gained can help doctors, within their own consultational styles, to better manage their interaction with patients. Plentiful clinical case vignettes illustrate this approach to understanding and managing clinical transactions and will be welcomed by clinical students and doctors in training, as well as by their trainers.

PROBLEMS WITH PATIENTS:
MANAGING COMPLICATED TRANSACTIONS

To our families and the friends
who supported our work.

PROBLEMS WITH PATIENTS: MANAGING COMPLICATED TRANSACTIONS

KINGSLEY NORTON

*Consultant Psychotherapist, Henderson Hospital, St Helier NHS Trust,
and Honorary Senior Lecturer, Section of Forensic Psychiatry,
Department of Mental Health Sciences, St George's Hospital Medical School, London*

SAM SMITH

*General Practitioner and General Practitioner Trainer,
Helsby Health Centre, Warrington*

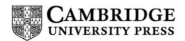

CAMBRIDGE
UNIVERSITY PRESS

Published by the Press Syndicate of the University of Cambridge
The Pitt Building, Trumpington Street, Cambridge CB2 1RP
40 West 20th Street, New York, NY 10011-4211, USA
10 Stamford Road, Oakleigh, Melbourne 3166, Australia

First published 1994

Printed in Great Britain at the University Press, Cambridge

A catalogue record for this book is available from the British Library

Library of Congress cataloguing in publication data

Norton, Kinglsey.
Problems with patients / Kingsley Norton and Sam Smith.
p.   cm.
Includes bibliographical references and index.
ISBN 0 521 43043 7 (hardback). – ISBN 0 521 43628 1 (pbk.)
1. Physician and patient.   I. Smith, Sam, 1951– .   II. Title.
[DNLM: 1. Physician–Patient Relations.   2. Attitude of Health
Personnel.   W62 N885p 1994]
R727.3.N67   1994
610.69′6 – dc20
DNLM/DLC for Library of Congress   93-33589 CIP

ISBN 0 521 43043 7   hardback
ISBN 0 521 43628 1   paperback

Contents

Foreword

I have spent more than forty years in clinical practice, nearly all of that time as a general practitioner. The arena in which I perform (compete?) as a general practitioner is the clinical consultation, and the environment in that arena depends upon the nature and quality of my relationship with each person who consults me. The study of the process of consultations and of the quality of doctor–patient relationships is, then, a proper occupation for any clinician, but most especially for a generalist. The motivation for undertaking such study is a pervasive sense of discomfort experienced by the empathic doctor who has just conducted an unsatisfactory (unsatisfying?) encounter with a patient. For the patient there is escape into the real world since his or her performance in consultation is not a professional obligation. As one humorist worded it: 'My doctor is nice; every time I see him I feel ashamed of what I think of doctors in general.'

As generation succeeds generation, the proper study of humans produces fresh theories and models to explain human behaviour in dyads and in groups large and small. Kingsley Norton and Sam Smith have taken human encounters and applied to them an appropriate range of new ideas and old. You may share in my experience of pleasure when I survive a difficult consultation without harming the patient or of dealing with my lack of satisfaction without being punitive to client or staff. If so you will find this book illuminating, rewarding, and instructive to read.

Professor Paul Freeling, O.B.E.

Preface

Certain patients are experienced by doctors as being particularly problematic, irrespective of the diagnosis or the inherent complexities of their medical condition. Somehow, with these individuals, the potentially straightforward process of the consultation and its outcome are adversely affected. Sometimes strong personal feelings are generated in doctor, patient or both. The transaction may become adversarial (even on occasion to the point of violence) with both parties increasingly locked into a stalemate from which clinical concerns are partially or totally excluded. Avoiding such clinically sterile interactions, by preventing the development of complicated clinical transactions, or successfully managing them, is in the interests of patients, doctors and the overall health care system. Doctors working in any clinical setting may be faced with patients whom they label as a 'difficult' or 'problem' patient. However, the doctor working in primary care is in an especially influential position acting, at least to an extent, as gatekeeper to the secondary tier of health care services. How he or she deals with complicated clinical transactions, and the extent to which such dealings are successful, will also determine how many and which patients are referred to the secondary tier.

Labelling patients as 'problems' represents, of course, a doctor-centred view. The real difficulty is more productively construed in terms of the interaction between doctor and patient as they perform their respective roles. This interaction is pursued within the context of the overall doctor–patient relationship, which, particularly in a primary care setting, can extend over many years and gain considerable significance in the lives of doctors and patients alike. The importance of the quality of this relationship is well recognised and has been extensively written about. The impact of its emotional and psychological aspects has the potential not only to enhance and support any necessary clinical work but also to subvert it. A common cause of difficulty, therefore, is the eruption of personal aspects of the doctor–patient interaction into their professional relationship. Such problems faced by doctors and patients formed the basis for informal discussions between the authors over a number of years. Indirectly, this book is the result.

As with many discussions, our ideas and arguments developed to include issues external to the clinical transaction: the practice or hospital clinic organisation, the health service as an entire system, implications for the training of doctors. However, the focus remains the doctor–patient interaction, albeit with an awareness of the social, emotional and physical context of the transaction. In particular, the emphasis is on the way in which often barely recognised, or even unconscious, emotional aspects of the personal level of the doctor–patient interaction can exert an influence that corrupts the straightforward process of the consultation and under-mines efforts to secure its legitimate goals. Negative feelings engendered by patients are sometimes difficult to acknowledge, since they may seem out of place in the mind of a professional carer. Sometimes their existence is entirely denied unless or until evidence is unwittingly produced to the contrary. It is therefore important that these aspects of the doctor–patient interaction are recognised. With practice, such emotional 'communi-cations' with the patient can be seen to have a meaning that can be understood, appreciated, and also provide valuable clues as to the source, and possible resolution, of the problem.

In order to understand such personal aspects of doctor and patient (especially those unconscious aspects) various strands of different theories are drawn together: social role theory, psychodynamic theory, and systems theory. The relevant concepts deriving from these theories are explained and applied to the clinical transaction between doctor and patient. Their application not only enhances an understanding of the complicated nature of the doctor–patient transaction, in dealings with so-called problem patients, but also suggests where and how interventions may be attempted in order to return the complicated transaction to the straightforward. Successful interventions often have the effect of reinforcing or buttressing the boundaries of legitimate clinical concerns.

Straightforward and complicated clinical transactions are defined in the book but neither represents a 'diagnosis' that can be concisely formulated. Having a clear notion of complicated clinical transactions, however, alerts the doctor to potentially disruptive influences or resultant departures from the straightforward, at the level of societal roles or of doctor and patient as unique individuals. Thus, complications may be identified early, while they are still relatively insignificant or minor and the chances of their being remedied are the greater. In this way, the sometimes gross caricatures of patients described in the literature ('heart-sink', 'hateful', 'fat folder' or 'thick chart', 'turkey') can potentially be avoided.

This book is not specifically concerned with treating psychological problems or psychiatric disorder, nor about developing counselling or psychotherapy skills. Its purpose is to help doctors to develop an attitude towards, and conceptualisation of, the clinical transactions with their patients that may prevent complicated (or preserve straightforward) clinical transactions. The approach complements rather than competes with others, such as problem-solving approaches, and does not constrain the doctor's usual style of consulting. Many doctors are already highly skilled in the areas of interviewing and clinical communication, often intuitively so. The aim of this book is to facilitate the management of complicated clinical transactions by introducing a methodical approach based on a theoretical underpinning which informs the choice of any intervention required. In particular, the method allows information derived from the personal level of the doctor–patient interaction to be harnessed in the service of the public level interaction and hence of the overall clinical transaction.

Increasingly, much of medical practice is recognised as being the result of a collaborative effort. Thus, in both primary and secondary care settings, the doctor is often but one member of a multi-disciplinary team. Much of what is said about the doctor–patient transaction, therefore, is also pertinent to transactions between other clinicians and their patients or clients. Doctor–doctor and other professional–professional non-clinical transactions can similarly be understood in the light of the concept of complicated transactions.

In Chapter 1, the arguments in favour of an interactive approach to the understanding of so-called 'problem patients' are rehearsed in the light of the relevant sociological and medical literature. In Chapter 2, straightforward and complicated clinical transactions are introduced as concepts and defined. Also, transaction and system 'windows' are introduced at this point as convenient shorthand devices for analysing a clinical transaction according to its public and personal domains and the external influences that impinge upon it. Chapters 3, 4 and 5 provide relevant psychodynamic and systems theory concepts, personality development, unconscious motivation, the effect of past relationships on the clinical transaction, those especially at risk of developing complicated clinical transactions, open systems, hierarchical and overlapping systems and isomorphy. Chapters 6 and 7 outline management strategies and interventions for managing complicated clinical transactions that derive from the conceptual model advanced earlier. Chapter 8 outlines the application of clinical transaction theory to the organisation and management of the clinical setting and is applicable to hospital outpatient clinics as well as to primary care settings. Finally, in Chapter 9, the implications for training doctors are considered, including the need to develop an appropriate attitude towards the doctor–patient interaction as well as knowledge and skills in recognising, analysing and dealing with complicated transactions. (Note: All the clinical examples quoted in the book are based on actual people and real encounters. However, key details have been altered so as to preserve anonymity.)

Two appendices are provided. The first augments Chapter 1 and describes some of the relevant phenomena in relation to complicated clinical transactions, but from the conventional doctor-centred perspective: somatisation, denial of physical illness, hysteria, hypochondriasis, alexithymia, Munchausen's syndrome, and malingering. The second provides information related to patients diagnosed as having personality disorder. This diagnosis is associated with sometimes profound difficulties in adopting an appropriate sick role. In addition, the personal level of interaction between such patients and their doctors may more readily yield factors capable of complicating the clinical transaction.

If after reading this book the reader, when next confronted with a patient who otherwise might be labelled as a 'problem', *first* reflects on what contribution he or she might be making to the complication, then we shall have achieved our main purpose. Any solutions to problems arising out of their interaction will derive from working *with* patients.

Kingsley Norton
Sam Smith

Acknowledgments

We are indebted to a great number of people for support and help with this book. Medical teachers at Clare College, Cambridge, and St George's Hospital Medical School inadvertently contributed by selecting us to train as doctors in the same student intake. Many other teachers subsequently have fostered our professional development and desire to communicate some of our own ideas and clinical experiences. A previous teacher and a number of current colleagues have made helpful and specific comments on a draft version of the book, namely: Professor A. H. Crisp, Drs Richard and Teresa Adair, Liz Agnew, Richard Brook, Chris Evans, John Formby, John Valentine, Jim Wilson and Ms Jan Wiener. Chris Norton provided a critical non-medical reading of earlier drafts and suggested numerous invaluable improvements to both style and content. Any remaining deficiencies in either area, however, remain essentially our own.

A special thanks must go to Ms Julia Wilding, who typed the very many drafts of this book with great patience and ever believing that the work would one day be completed. We are also very grateful to Professor Paul Freeling for kindly agreeing to provide a Foreword to our book. We approached him out of respect for his own contribution to the field of clinical consultation, which we, like him, believe to be central to the practice of all branches of medicine.

1

Doctor–patient interaction

> The best kind of patient ... is one who from great suffering
> and danger of life or sanity responds quickly to a treatment
> that interests his doctor and thereafter remains completely well;
> but those who recover only slowly or incompletely are less
> satisfying.
>
> Dr Tom Main (1957)

Introduction

Mr Taylor entered the consulting room almost stealthily and took his seat. The doctor's greeting was received silently with a somewhat jeering smile. Mr Taylor had a shifty appearance, accentuated by the wandering of his gaze, which was hardly ever allowed to engage the doctor's. He began to detail his minor complaints, which were numerous. The doctor, looking at his own notes, saw uncomfortably that Mr Taylor was regularly prescribed five different medications, three of which might potentially interact in a harmful way. As he listened, endeavouring to make contact with Mr Taylor's wandering gaze, the doctor's shoulders drooped as if in resignation. From long experience he sensed nothing would change as a result of this clinical encounter. Mr Taylor left with a prescription to continue all five drugs, a prescription written guiltily and received with an almost sadistic smile, the only steady eye contact of the consultation.

The above clinical vignette based on an actual doctor–patient interaction (videotaped and discussed by trainer and trainee) represents a consultation with which most doctors are familiar. Mr Taylor is a so-called 'problem patient'. He does not appear to experience great suffering and certainly does not have a life-threatening disease. In spite of repeated consultations little progress is made in alleviating his multiple complaints. The doctor's initial interest and hope that cure or amelioration might be forthcoming becomes replaced by an increasing sense of pessimism, frustration, guilt and hopelessness.

However, doctors vary in whom they describe as problem patients and such patients are variously labelled 'self-pitiers' (Hackett, 1969), 'crocks' (Lipsitt, 1970), 'obnoxious' (Martin, 1975), 'unpopular' (Stockwell, 1984), 'familiar face' or 'fat folders' (Schrire, 1986), 'heart-sink'

1

(O'Dowd, 1988), as well as hysterics, hypochondriacs and malingerers. What characterises such groupings and how much they may overlap is unclear.

In an early report, four categories of 'hateful patients' were defined (Groves, 1978). The author suggested that it was the insatiable dependency of such patients that led to the four behavioural stereotypes that he described. The 'dependent clinger' expresses excessive thanks and gratitude for actions taken by the doctor but also constantly seeks repeated reassurance for minor problems. The 'entitled demander' appears to view the doctor as a barrier to receiving services and constantly complains to Health Authorities about imagined shortcomings in the services received. The 'manipulative help-rejecter' presents a series of symptoms the doctor is powerless to improve. Finally, there is the 'self-destructive denier', for example the patient with severe vascular disease who refuses even to consider giving up smoking. The importance of acknowledging negative feelings evoked by such patients is particularly stressed by the author, since this emotional aspect of the doctor's response is considered to constitute important clinical information, useful in managing these patients.

Another approach to the classification of problem patients resulted in the identification of six subtypes, expressed as caricatures: the listmaker, the actress or actor, the demanding one, the helpless one, the doubting Thomas, and the up and down personality (Roukeema, 1976). Gaining confidence in managing these differing personality types is seen to be a key factor in enabling doctors to perceive such patients as a challenge rather than the reason for having a 'bad day' on their account.

Others have produced different categorisations of problem patients, for example masked depressives, seekers of secondary gain, and those with the 'tired person' syndrome (Jarvis, 1987). This classification introduced the tired person syndrome, which is viewed as a common variant of problem patient often overlooked in clinical practice. Such patients tend to be either older people who have demonstrable organic disease or else younger people who suddenly undergo a crisis that decreases their level of functioning. All apparently demonstrate a real or perceived loss of function and productivity that is accompanied by loss of self-esteem. The decrease in self-esteem is thought to trigger anxiety, which may be severe. A vicious circle becomes established. Treatment, which is acknowledged to be difficult, involves the doctor 'accepting and legitimising the very real loss that the patient perceives in order to help him or her become comfortably dependent' (Jarvis, 1987).

Another descriptive approach to the classification of problem patients, emphasising the importance of the doctor–patient interaction, suggests three main types: the stubborn, obdurate patient; the manipulative or seductive patient; and the violent and sometimes paranoid patient (Smith and Steindler, 1983). Smith and Steindler offer useful tips on the management of these patients, including how doctors might best withstand the impact of such patients. They comment on ways of preventing burn-out in professionals, problem patients being viewed as contributing to this outcome. Among the strategies recommended is communicating and collaborating with peers and with supervisors over difficult clinical problems.

Others have recommended a long case meeting, with multi-disciplinary staff, to discuss difficult patients (Gerrard and Riddell, 1988). These authors identified ten categories of such patients, which they briefly defined with case examples, together with suggested ways to understand and 'unlock patient and (a) doctor'. Of their ten categories, they singled out two, 'black holes' and 'secrets', for special mention. Black holes refer to patients who demand help persistently but who are also expert in blocking it. With regard to such patients, their conclusion was a negative one, namely that time would often be better spent on other patients. The category of 'secrets' refers to families that on family interview were found to have a secret that had lain untold for many years. The authors commented that family interviews became increasingly part of their everyday practice.

From the above, it can be seen that doctors subjectively use the term 'problem patient' to label a variety of patients. Such patients present with vague and shifting symptoms involving multiple organ systems, chronically complain, constantly worry about their health and contribute in other ways to their doctor's uncertainty and frustration (McGaghie and Whitenack, 1982). Little work has been undertaken to measure reliably doctors' perceptions of the degree to which individuals display problem patient characteristics but, in the paper just cited, the authors described the use of a scale they devised to measure doctors' subjective clinical impressions. They view the labelling process of problem patients as involving the doctors' interpretation of a complex set of 'biomedical, demographic and psychosocial data' and believe that their Patient Description Questionnaire measure shows promise.

There appear to be no sufficiently distinct attributes of problem patients that distinguish a single homogeneous grouping (McGaghie and Whitenack, 1982). Such patients tend to seek far more medical care than average (von Mering and Earley, 1966). They have communication difficulties with their physicians and tend to be unco-operative and poor historians with few objective findings and an unusually large number of complaints and demands, and are also more likely than others to be referred to secondary care specialists (Corney *et al.*, 1988). Partly because of this and because such patients tend to have more psychiatric symptoms, psychiatrists have studied some problem patients in depth. Often there has been little precision or consistency in the psychiatric and psychological terminology applied but certain phenomena relevant to a consideration of problem patients have emerged. These tend to transcend conventional diagnostic categories but still represent a doctor-centred perspective. They include somatisation, denial of physical illness, hysteria, hypochondriasis, alexithymia, Munchausen's syndrome, and malingering. (See Appendix I for a discussion of these aspects.)

Perhaps unsurprisingly, problem patients compared with non-problem patients score more highly on scales relating to adverse health beliefs and psychological dysfunction (Whitenack and McGaghie, 1984). This fact in itself, however, cannot adequately account for the often pejorative use of the terms doctors use when describing problem patients. Such descriptions are stigmatic labels and it seems likely that doctors' negative feelings towards such patients underpin and fuel the labelling process. These labels may result, at least in part, from the fact that problem patients often appear not to play their role, as patients, in the way in which their doctors expect them to. The doctor in such a situation may well feel a sense of frustration, failure or impotence. Such feelings may be acknowledged with an effort made to understand what they symbolise within the doctor–patient relationship. Alternatively, doctors may respond by minimising, disowning or reacting to their feelings unthinkingly. Furthermore, the patient may be blamed for the feelings. When this happens, it is as if the patient is held totally responsible for generating the doctor's discomfort. What began as a professional encounter, with more or less discrete clinical goals, is in danger of becoming little more than a clash of personalities. Not only does this adversely affect the process and quality of the consultation but it threatens the attainment of clinical goals. Such a disturbed state of affairs may continue unacknowledged or perhaps an uncomfortable stalemate ensues, in which both doctor and patient attribute blame or faults to the other. Alternatively the relationship breaks down altogether. In any event, the appropriate clinical work will prove both hard-going and unrewarding. If, however, doctors accept that in their interaction with certain patients their perception of them is influenced by their own anger, irritation or disappointment, then it becomes clear that both patients and doctors play their part in generating the stigmatic label 'problem patient'. On this account, it has been argued that the doctor–patient interaction itself should be the focus of any attempt to understand more fully what constitues the concept of the problem patient. In this sense it is not patients who are problematic but doctors' dealings with them (Schuller, 1977; Kuch *et al.*, 1977; Groves, 1978).

To gain more understanding of the doctor–patient interaction, it is necessary to examine those factors that determine the doctor's and patient's expectations of each other. As a first step in this endeavour, it is useful to divide the doctor–patient interaction, albeit arbitrarily, into public and personal domains. These public and personal domains constitute differing conceptual levels. Expectations arising in the public domain may be seen as deriving from the attributes of the socially structured roles of doctor and patient. Conversely, those expectations arising in the personal domain derive from the idiosyncratic mix of attributes that go to make up doctor and patient as individual people. It is important to bear in mind, however, that in practice public and personal domains may be difficult to distinguish and that they interact.

The public domain

The public level of interaction between patient and doctor is shaped, moulded and confined by the pressure to conform to the social roles 'doctor' and 'patient'. Roles are those parts of individual and group behaviour that are defined by society and social structure. They define what is socially acceptable and what is socially deviant. Their influence on behaviour acts to reinforce social norms and expectations and, by setting the boundaries of social interaction, they place constraints on idiosyncratic or impulsive behaviour (Turner, 1962).

Stereotypes and stigmatic labelling

By conforming to socially predefined roles, behaviour becomes predictable. The stereotype 'doctor' might include those attributes of a caring, interested and helpful expert, with powers to restore the patient to health and minimise suffering. Such a positive stereotype is image-enhancing and therefore likely to be acceptable to most doctors. Needless to say, however, not all stereotypes are image-enhancing and the negative stereotype of the 'problem patient' can be a stigmatising label.

Stigmatic labelling, as a process, has important implications for the doctor–patient interaction and, of course, it operates in both directions to create the 'problem patient' or the 'quack'. In the process, the whole person is redefined, not just those aspects that may have engendered the label. When applied, the result is a more or less subtle shift of attention away from the main concern (i.e. the reason for the consultation) toward what is now perceived as the deviance of the patient or doctor. As a consequence, the person may no longer be perceived and responded to as the original 'whole'. The label comes to define, thus, the entire personality, so that any remaining personal attributes become tainted, blemished or discounted. Once labelled as 'problem', patients' identities are, in effect, distorted, with a wide range of imperfections attributed to them.

The label 'problem' thus stigmatises the patient. However, in its effect it does much more than this. The doctor's ability to sustain the role of doctor in the doctor–patient interaction, especially in primary care settings, depends in great measure on an ability to empathise with the patient and identify with the patient's predicament (see Chapter 4). However careful the doctor may be, once the stigmatising level has become established, the doctor's capacity for empathy or even sympathy is diminished. In the process the doctor becomes disempowered. By focussing on the stigmatised attributes of patients, their 'stupidity' or 'hypochondriasis', doctors place their patients out of professional reach because the valid medical task the patients present is relegated in importance, ignored or avoided. When this happens, doctors run the risk of disowning all or part of the responsibility that they bear for their patients by virtue of their social role as doctor.

Conversely, when patients stigmatically label their doctors, they are unlikely to heed advice or entrust themselves appropriately to their doctors' care. Stigmatic labels therefore may be applied to both doctor and patient in their respective roles. Unpleasant personal confrontation may result and can escalate to the point where clinical goals are lost sight of altogether. When this happens the long-term worth of the doctor–patient relationship becomes seriously, sometimes irretrievably, compromised.

Although social roles imply stereotypes, and hence are vulnerable to the process of stigmatic labelling, they also serve the valuable function of defining limits to the professional relationship of doctor and patient. They strongly influence therefore what patients might legitimately ask of their doctors and what doctors might be expected to deliver in response. The doctor's role can be a very difficult one to perform, including as sometimes it may, elements of social worker, priest, policeman and psychoanalyst. It is not without its limits, however, and every doctor will know what it feels like to be pushed to or beyond those limits. It is often at such times, when doctors feel that more is being demanded of them than they can, or perhaps should, deliver, that patients become labelled as 'problems'.

The role of doctor

By virtue of medical training, and often almost incidental to it, medical students develop into doctors who are capable of entering into professional relationships with their patients. That is to say, they acquire the ability to perform the social role of doctor within the public domain. This transformation equips fully fledged doctors with the attitudes, skills and knowledge that enable them, on the one hand, to maintain a certain degree of detachment from their patients, yet on the other hand to remain in sympathetic, if not empathic, contact. Such a professional stance maximises the likelihood of an objective assessment of the patient and his or her illness and, at the same time, encourages the trust and co-operation necessary for successful treatment.

There is little consensus in the literature on the subject of the significance and relevance of the doctor's consultation style, a fact that may stem from the absence of a coherent model and theoretical framework (Pendleton, 1983). Certainly there are difficulties inherent in deriving theoretical models that hold good for all illnesses, patients and doctors. Nevertheless, evidence of the importance of the doctor's style is reflected in the growing interest, particularly in primary care settings, in the acquisition of interviewing and counselling skills.

It is asserted by some observers that doctors assume different models of doctor–patient relationships to suit given circumstances (Szasz and Hollender, 1956). On the contrary, it is claimed that doctors develop a stock set of behaviour patterns that are applied generally regardless of the nature of the presenting problem (Byrne and Long, 1976). Doctors have been noted to display a degree of flexibility in assuming different roles in relation to patients with alcohol, as opposed to opiate, usage (Roche *et al.*, 1991). Overall, however, the doctors in this study seemed to conform to patterns of three broad groupings, namely interactive problem-solvers, traditionalist healers, and technologists. For the purposes of this study, the definitions of the typology were as follows: the interactive problem-solver plays a collaborative role in a wide range of prevention, maintenance and disease issues and incorporates conselling with technical medical skills; traditionalist healers see their role as doctor primarily in disease-related issues that involve some listening skills but basically they retain an 'instructor' outlook; expert technologists see their roles as primarily concerned with the physical sequelae of illness and their expertise lies in the clinical management of disease rather than in the management of the whole person. The conclusion from the study was that doctors' responses could be seen to lie along dimensions that encompass factors such as attitudes to technology, model of medical practice assumed and interpersonal variables.

Other typologies have been suggested. For example, doctors have been construed as being along two dimensions – scientific orientation and social orientation – and forming four groups (Mechanic, 1970): moderns, counsellors, withdrawers, and technicians. A large survey of 2104 general practitioners lent some support to the above typology (Calnan, 1988). No comprehensive typologies, however, have become securely established. For example, as a result of a cluster analytic technique to examine doctors' responses to questions on their prescribing and referral behaviour, five groups of doctors have been proposed: egalitarian, traditional, old style, doctor-centred, and patient-centred (Bucks *et al.*, 1990).

The effect of age has been studied in relation to the doctor's style. Mechanic's study, cited above, indicated a relatively large number of young doctors in the group labelled 'technicians'. In Calnan's study, however, it was found that doctors tending to have a social orientation were more likely to be under thirty-five years of age. Likewise, Bucks and colleagues found that the most conservative group, the 'old stylers', comprised older doctors. Interpreting these conflicting results is clearly problematic. It has been suggested, none the less, that the greater social orientation of younger doctors may reflect merely characteristics of youthfulness, with clinicians becoming more conservative and less flexible with increasing age and experience (Abed and Neira-Muñoz, 1990). The absence of adequate longitudinal studies to test these alternative explanations means that this question, which has important implications for medical education, remains unanswered.

The significance of the doctor's style, as an influence on the outcome of the patient's treatment, is poorly understood. Perhaps unsurprisingly, there is accumulating evidence that the quality of doctor–patient communication relates to a patient's sense of satisfaction (Horder and Moore, 1990). The doctor's style of consultation has also been shown to influence patient satisfaction, particularly in those presenting with physical problems and those receiving a prescription (Savage and Armstrong, 1990).

During medical training, emphasis is on the teaching and learning of disease entities. Skills are demonstrated and knowledge imparted so that the diseased and the non-diseased can be differentiated. Initially, the approach tends to be, to an extent, theoretical and reductive and must be so in order to serve the purpose of the diagnostic endeavour. A certain distancing and detachment from the patient is, therefore, both necessary and desirable. But for many students embarking on training, the notion of becoming a doctor appeals because of the idea of a therapeutic relationship between two people – the doctor and the patient – as opposed to a relationship solely between the doctor and the patient's illness (see Balint, 1957). The problem remains of how to establish a relationship that not only allows an objective assessment of the patient's illness (public domain activity) but at the same time maintains the patient's integrity so that the relationship is between two real people (personal domain). The public and personal levels of the doctor–patient interaction do not always harmonise and at times there may be considerable dissonance between them.

The medical model

The medical model of disease has long been the basic paradigm of medicine following the development of the germ theory of disease in the nineteenth century. It remains the principal form of explanation in scientific medicine. Its fundamental assumptions can be stated as follows (Abercrombie *et al.*, 1984). First, all disease is caused by a specific agent (the 'disease entity'), such as a virus, parasite or bacterium. Second, the patient is to be regarded as the passive target of medical intervention, since scientific medicine is concerned with the body as a sort of machine, rather than with a person in a complex social environment. Third, restoring health requires the use of medical technology and advanced scientific procedures.

While being eclipsed, especially in primary care and preventive medicine, this view of disease continues to underpin much of medical practice and particularly so in hospital medicine. Doctors will obviously vary in the extent to which their own professional style and practice derives from a rigid adherence to the principles of the medical model. Although few may recognise themselves as the implied caricature that stems from the fundamental assumptions of the model, it appears that doctors can be differentiated, at least to some extent, according to their doctor-centredness and their use of medical technology. How usefully the medical model can be applied in the interests of an individual patient will depend upon, among other things, how classical is the illness presented. In an uncomplicated case of a patient complaining of symptoms that are correctly diagnosed as due to a disease with a recognised physical cause and proven pharmacological or surgical remedy, the model fits quite well. Other factors being equal, the doctor's style or ability to communicate with the patient may be of only marginal significance. The further the patient's presenting complaint or illness deviates from the classical, however, the more the doctor's style will influence the process and outcome of treatment. Ideally, doctors should be able to adapt their styles to suit the requirements of their patients and the patients' illnesses, taking into account the effects of any treatment and the influence of, and impact on, the patients' wider psychological and social environments.

The role of patient

Ideally, patients present their illnesses in a manner that elicits a reciprocal professional response from the doctor. Thus, the patient makes a timely presentation of a genuine illness that is accurately diagnosed and appropriately treated. In such an instance, the normal expectations each has of the other, by virtue of their respective social roles, are realised in a straightforward way. The patient's 'illness behaviour' (Mechanic, 1962), however, is not learned in the same way as the doctor's professional behaviour. There is no equivalent scientific body of knowledge underpinning symptoms from the patient's perspective. (This remains true even though the general population is increasingly enlightened in respect of medical matters, largely through the media's reporting of medical advances.) Indeed, symptoms may not be experienced as the discrete entities implied by the terms patients use to describe them.

Mr Allen, a young man in his early twenties, complained of feeling 'tired and weak'. He denied other symptoms, and physical examination revealed no obvious abnormality, specifically no loss of power. Further clarification of the complaint showed that the man was depressed and hopeless in mood. This was related to his having been recently passed over for promotion at work. Previously he had tended to be a shy and meticulous person with few interests outside of his job. Other features, for example insomnia, that might have suggested a diagnosis of depressive disorder were absent. On closer questioning, it was found that Mr Allen's sense of energy was lowered but that he maintained a full range of activities and, in fact, he was not actually more tired than usual nor was he weaker. The terms 'tired' and 'weak' referred to his emotional state.

Informal 'training' for the patient's role is acquired from the immediate family and wider social network. Patients' social contexts powerfully influence the way in which they construe illness and seek medical help (Herzlich, 1975; Blaxter, 1983). Illness-related beliefs, the language used in response to it or in description of illness, and even the body language for distress, are all, to an extent, a reflection of the social class and culture to which individuals and their families belong (Lipowski, 1988). Families themselves may exhibit habitual responses to illness. Research suggests that children exposed to physical illness and displays of pain in other family members may somatise more as adults, perhaps through processes of identification and modelling. Thus, it is often important for the doctor openly and directly to explore the patient's health beliefs and attitudes, since they may have considerable bearing on the timing and mode of presentation of symptoms, the acceptability of treatment or advice and the patient's expectations of health care in general.

Mrs North had been seeing her doctor regularly following an episode of acute pericarditis. At the time she had been quite seriously ill and afterwards she remained anxious and depressed. Initially, her doctor understood this as a reaction to her life-threatening illness. It was only after many months that it became clear her persistent anxiety was associated with agoraphobia. She was protected from having to deal with her agoraphobia by her family, especially by her daughter, who frequently took on mother's tasks both within the house and outside of it, for example doing all the shopping for her mother. As the tangle of family relationships was explored, Mrs North was persuaded that her agoraphobia was something for which she could legitimately seek help and she was referred to a clinical psychologist with whom she made considerable progress.

In this instance it appeared that it was Mrs North's difficulty with asking for help that lay behind her full recovery from her pericarditis. She believed that her psychological difficulties should have been within her own control and consequently she was ashamed to admit them. Her family's initial support for her, and especially the action taken by her daughter, turned into obstacles to her full social and psychological recovery. These obstacles were removed only once a full airing of the issues had taken place and after referral to the secondary level of care.

Personality and personality disorder

Each person's illness is unique. Everyone reacts to disease and its implications, and to the effects and implications of any treatment, with an individual style (Kahana and Bibring, 1965). This important fact, which in some ways undermines the potency of the medical model of illness, forms the basis of the maxim 'treat the patient, not the disease'. The patient's illness is the result of the complex interaction between the disease and its treatment, the relationship (by virtue of status as a patient) with the doctor and the relationship between personality and wider psycho-social contexts. The outcome of this interaction will in important ways determine patient's behaviour in the face of illness (Chesser, 1975; see Figure 1.1).

Some patients may seek to avoid coming to terms with illness by partially or totally withdrawing from treatment or defaulting from follow-up. Others may freeze or capitulate, becoming passive to the extent of being unable to participate actively even in essential treatment or

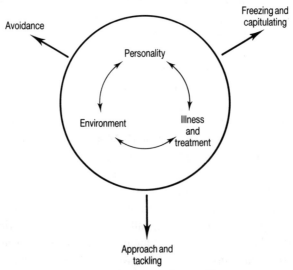

Figure 1.1. Patients' reaction to illness.

rehabilitation. Others may approach and tackle illness, sufficiently adjusting their lives, temporarily or permanently, so as to minimise the risks to health. When illness poses what is perceived as an overwhelming threat to wellbeing, coping strategies may become intensified to the point of gross disturbances of behaviour. Florid neurotic reactions, psychosis or even suicide may be the result. In any event, clinically significant depression commonly accompanies physical illness. Often, the illness signifies to the patient a loss – anatomical, functional or symbolic (Parkes, 1975).

Psychiatric illness and abnormal personality (whether or not amounting to personality disorder) hamper a patient's adaptation to illness (Appendix II). Anxious patients usually become more anxious and sometimes also hypochondriacal, irritable, hostile or unco-operative. Those with a dependent personality, who may be model patients while their needs are met, become overdemanding of care, time, support and explanation when frustrated. The histrionic patient, too, when ill may demand much of the doctor's attention. Obsessional personalities find adaptation to change especially difficult and tend to react to unexpected changes of management with high levels of anxiety. Those with aggressive, antisocial, paranoid or schizoid personalities tend to become more so under the stress induced by physical illness. Physical illness may precipitate relapse of psychiatric illnesses such as manic-depressive psychosis or schizophrenia.

Problems associated with managing patients with personality disorder (APA, 1987; WHO, 1992) to some extent represent an extension of the above. However, personality disordered patients are discussed in this book in terms of their habitual deployment of immature psychological defence mechanisms that tend to set up a particular style of interaction (infantile dependent) in relation to the doctors with whom they come into professional contact (see Chapters 3, 4 and Appendix II). Also important is the influence of the doctor's personality and any abnormalities of it, again whether or not amounting to personality disorder.

The sick role and abnormal illness behaviour

In the straightforward clinical transaction both the patient and the doctor play their complementary social roles, as patient and doctor. In this respect the notion of the 'sick role' (Parsons, 1951) is of value in so far as it represents the granting of permission to patients to behave in ways that, were the patients not sick, would be deemed unacceptable. The sick role has four main features. First, the sick person is exempt from normal social role responsibilities. Second, the sick person cannot be expected to get better by an act of decision or will. Third, the sick person has an obligation to want to get well. Fourth, the sick person has an obligation, depending on the severity of the condition, to seek technically competent help, usually via a doctor, and furthermore to co-operate with the doctor in the process of getting well. Many, although by no means all, patients are able to play their part, as patients, appropriately. By so doing they make the task of the doctors, in carrying out their own social role, relatively straightforward, even though the diagnostic and treatment challenges may be considerable.

The concept of the sick role, however, has been criticised, not least because it allows little room for conflicting interest, aims, views or explanations between patient and doctor (Freidson, 1970). It is obvious that patients do not consult doctors for every symptom they experience. However, it is not easy to explain, at least according to the rationality of the medical model, why patients with symptoms but without disease should choose to consult their doctors. Within 'medical rationality', the symptom, as a manifestation of disease, cannot exist independently. That there are such patients who persist in reporting symptoms to their doctors, despite the reassurance of 'a reasonably lucid explanation' that there is no defective pathology present, has given rise to the concept of abnormal illness behaviour (Pilowsky, 1969). This concept reflects a rather narrow perspective whereby symptoms without disease are 'as impossible as flames without fire' (Armstrong, 1986).

It is obvious that the patient's encounter with the doctor does not necessarily represent a cosy reciprocity of roles. Within medical sociology, therefore, newer explanatory models of illness behaviour have developed that stress that the meeting between the doctor and patient is essentially problematic and certainly warranting of close scrutiny (Armstrong, 1986). Patient-centred sociological studies have sought to ask patients them-selves for their own subjective reports as to why they did (or did not) present symptoms to a doctor (Robinson, 1971). Findings from this line of research have proved revealing. Patients do not tend to present their symptoms passively for interpretation and explanation by the doctor. Rather, they already have their own more or less well-developed constructs to evaluate and account for bodily feelings prior to consultation. In this sense, they do not present symptoms but a 'theory' of their illness. Although it may not accord with medical learning, patients make reasoned decisions about self-medication or the use of alternative therapies of various sorts. Such non-medical and sometimes idiosyncratic logic may underpin non-compliance with treatment or account for the patient's frustration in what is perceived as the irrationality of so-called 'medical rationality' (Armstrong, 1986).

The implication of these findings is that if patients respond to illness in terms of their own lay theories, increasingly well informed, then their doctors cannot remain simply concerned with traditional diagnosis and treatment and the limits and constraints imposed by such an approach or style. Good clinical practice, therefore, calls for doctors to elicit, consider and respond to their patients' theories of illness (health beliefs), if outcome criteria such as satisfaction and compliance are to be improved.

The personal domain

The world of social roles, and of the public level of the doctor–patient interaction, is relatively static. The expectations of patients and doctors, within a given and stable society, tend to vary only a little with the passage of time. What change there is tends to take place by slow evolution. Within the personal domain, by contrast, the interaction between patient and doctor is potentially in a continuous state of flux. In order to be of value here, conceptual models applied must accommodate such a dynamic state of affairs.

The nature of the doctor–patient interaction, at the personal level, is that of a provider of care, in the form of medical advice, treatment or support, to a receiver of the same. Those attracted to medicine, as a career that embodies this dynamic giving–receiving relationship, have personal attributes that, while varied, probably represent a fairly narrow and distinct grouping. They may be contrasted to those attracted to, for example, the armed forces, the Church, or industrial management. Drawing a caricature: a doctor may be someone who wishes to make a contribution to society by helping the sick. To this end doctors accurately diagnose, appropriately treat and ultimately cure their grateful patients.

While some medical practice does actually tally with this simplistic view, often it will not. It is well recognised that diagnosis and treatment, at times, may be more art than science. Patients may not be cured and may not feel grateful! Inasmuch as doctors are drawn to medicine by an inner, personal need to 'give', and for others to receive gratefully, they will suffer disappointment to the extent that their contacts with patients fall short of this ideal, as sometimes they inevitably must. In so far as they do fall short, the quality of the interaction with patients will be diminished.

There is always, therefore, the potential for a significant blow to a doctor's self-esteem or self-confidence when diagnoses are missed or treatment fails to effect cure or symptomatic relief. If doctors find particular difficulty in tolerating such failure, then their own disappointment may well become a complicating factor within the interaction with their patients. Moreover, should patients detect this disappointment, they may themselves react adversely to it, especially, if they have difficulty asking for or receiving help. The scene is then set for the personal level of the interaction to surface, sometimes completely submerging the public level. The potential for this to happen is always present, and is testimony to the relative fragility of the public level interaction and the difficulty involved in performing and sustaining the appropriate social roles. It also serves to emphasise the dynamic nature of the doctor–patient interaction as a whole.

Doctors' needs to give and patients' capacities to seek or receive help are largely moulded by early familial relationships, in particular the relationship with their parents or parent substitutes (see Chapter 3). Doctors, for example, vary in the extent to which they can sustain professional (or other) disappointment without reacting by blaming others – the 'system', the Government, the patient or subordinate staff! Such reactions, mostly unwitting, may remain outside awareness, and their motivation partly or entirely unconscious. However, from the patient's point of view, they may be both obvious and unhelpful. A psychodynamic perspective allows the unconscious aspects of personality, often adversely influential in the doctor–patient relationships, to be considered. This is described in detail in Chapters 3 and 4.

The doctor–patient interaction is pursued within a 'system' (see Chapter 5) comprising the doctor and the patient. From governmental departments downwards, health services as a whole can be conceived of as hierarchies of systems, having as their base (at the interface with the society that it serves) the doctor–patient system. Changes in health service policy affect both health service staff and patients. Furthermore, they may be sudden in onset and dramatic in their impact (Norton *et al.*, 1992). The doctor–patient system, as the final common pathway, tends to bear and express the brunt of such changes. Accommodating a Government's policy changes, therefore, may strain the doctor–patient interaction if the impact of change is sudden and demands a rapid, reciprocal change in the doctor or patient role (as when the patient, for example, becomes a 'customer' as opposed to a 'grateful recipient'). This imposed strain on the interaction will inevitably find expression, to some degree, at the personal level. Thus changes instituted by the highest systems in the hierarchy feed downwards to affect many or all of their subsystems. This becomes problematic if the goals of the higher systems are not consonant with the goals of the subsystems. This theme is developed in later chapters.

Conclusions

There is a growing consensus among clinicians and theoreticians (especially those social scientists interested in the field of medicine) that:

(1) there is a subgroup of patients who are considered difficult to manage by virtue of factors other than the intrinsic complexity of their actual physical or psychological disorder;
(2) all doctor–patient interactions are potentially problematic;
(3) the doctor plays a role in the promotion or maintenance of the problematic interaction;
(4) the doctor's style, especially with respect to communication with the patient, correlates with outcome (at least in some instances);
(5) in the management of problem patients, specific strategies can usefully be deployed, taking into account, and if necessary involving, other people important in the patient's life;
(6) management plans should be construed with respect to the needs of the particular doctor–patient interaction;
(7) formal discussion with colleagues about the management of problem patients can be beneficial.

However, there is no comprehensive or coherent theoretical framework that might aid the doctor's understanding and inform consequent interventions in the management of problematic interactions with patients. What is required, therefore, is a model that can be applied by the doctor to *all* patients regardless of their presenting problems and that takes into account not only the patient as a unique individual but also the relevant wider psychosocial and cultural contexts. Moreover, such a model should permit a perspective that helps the doctor to identify difficulties in the interaction no matter how these are expressed, for example via treatment failure, poor compliance or frayed tempers. Ideally, such a perspective would help the doctor to avoid inadvertently contributing to the promotion or maintenance of an impaired doctor–patient relationship, bringing in its wake poor communication, patient and doctor dissatisfaction and, in many instances, a poor clinical outcome. This is particularly important since there is, overall, no consensus as to what categorises so-called problem patients both in terms of clinical and sociodemographic characteristics. Even though many problem patients do have 'fat folders' or 'thick charts' the latter start out thin!

The doctor–patient interaction is carried on in two domains, the public and the personal. These represent contrasting conceptual levels of the interaction. The influence of personal factors, on both patient and doctor, may render the performance of the social roles of doctor and patient problematic. Doctors, as 'givers', for their own personal reasons, may have difficulty when their 'gifts' are not gratefully received by their patients. Patients may experience difficulty in securing help, either because they find it hard to ask for, or have difficulty receiving it, or both. The impact of patients' illnesses may also strain their capacity to function psychologically and socially.

Doctors' and patients' expectations of one another tend to be relatively stable, although not immutable. Strain is induced, however, by changes, not only in the individual patient or doctor, but in the many systems of which they find themselves members. So long as the goals and responsibilities entailed by membership of each system do not conflict, the doctor–patient interaction as the final common pathway has no extra stress applied to it, i.e. the doctor and patient can simply and straightforwardly proceed with the relevant clinical work. When goals are incompatible, however, the scene is set for problems, and the potential for personal aspects to dominate is increased. The public level interaction, and the sustaining of social role responsibilities, are threatened if the quality of the personal level of the doctor–patient interaction is adversely affected. The result may be the stigmatic labelling of patients thereby placing them out of professional reach. The securing of clinical goals will be jeopardised as a consequence. Three different perspectives, sociological, psychodynamic, and systemic, aid an understanding of the complexity of the interaction between doctor and patient. These perspectives are discussed more fully in the rest of this book.

2

The clinical transaction

Introduction

Mrs Black, a mother of three children and a part-time telephonist, developed a painful throat and swollen glands during the course of an evening. She had a headache and fever, for which she took paracetamol. The next day her symptoms were more severe and, unable to work, she decided to consult her doctor, making an appointment to do so. When Mrs Black was seen and examined, the doctor, who knew her well and liked her, diagnosed acute tonsillitis and, communicating this to her, prescribed an appropriate antibiotic. Mrs Black complied with this treatment and recovered over the next few days.

This simple vignette is a common enough example of a clinical transaction in primary care with an outcome satisfactory to both doctor and patient. The term 'clinical transaction' is introduced here to refer specifically to the two-person, interactive system of doctor and patient. It embraces both the public and personal domains of their interaction. To 'transact' means: 'to carry through negotiations: to have dealings; do business; to treat; to manage or settle affairs' (*Shorter Oxford English dictionary*). A clinical transaction, therefore, is defined as: *an appropriately negotiated, goal-orientated interaction between doctor and patient, comprising both public and personal components.*

The process of the clinical transaction, considered as a negotiation, implies that patient and doctor share a more equal status than that of the traditionally portrayed doctor–patient interaction, even if certain inequalities remain. This differs from the traditional conception of the consultation, wherein the patient is regarded as a relatively passive recipient of advice or treatment. Thus, within the clinical transaction, the patient too is accorded a certain status of expert. This applies at least in

19

so far as knowledge and experience of the patient's own illness and personal difficulties are concerned.

Defined thus, the term 'clinical transaction' emphasises the interactive aspects of the doctor–patient relationship and goes some way toward avoiding the obstacles posed by an approach that places the patient as the sole object of study and as the source of any problem encountered by the doctor. As a consequence, problems are located in the transaction, rather than just in the patient or doctor. Also, the fact that the clinical transaction is goal-oriented places limits on the expectations of both patient and doctor. The implication is that, ideally, the doctor should deal with the problem as presented by the patient or else negotiate and agree an alternative agenda with the patient. In so doing, both doctor and patient are enabled to fulfil their social role responsibilities.

The ability of doctors to maintain and be aware of their part in the public interaction (i.e. their professional role) with their patients is crucial. Implicit is their capacity to recognise when the boundaries of the public domain of the clinical transaction are being crossed, extended, stretched or in some way undermined. This is likely to occur when personal factors overwhelm the public level interaction. Ideally, doctors' training and experience help them to contain their emotional shock, anxiety or disgust in response to their patients' disease, which were it too obvious might alarm or shame the patient. In most clinical encounters, however, the disease or illness is not so immediately threatening and responses on the personal level may be subtle. Such responses relate to the qualities of doctor and patient as people and may pass unnoticed or be dismissed as clinically unimportant. However, personal factors may have far-reaching implications for the quality of the doctor–patient relationship itself and, thereby, for the securing of clinical goals. If noticed and acknowledged, however, personal factors (i.e. attendant thoughts, feelings, attitudes and behaviours) that may come to dominate the doctor–patient interaction can function as important clues not only to problems within the inter-action but also to their solution. This theme is developed in later chapters (see especially Chapter 6).

Clinical transactions

Most clinical transactions are carried out in an atmosphere of mutual respect, clinical goals being secured as the result of an appropriate effort from both doctor and patient as in the case of Mrs Black, above. This situation may apply regardless of the reason for the patient consulting the doctor and irrespective of the illness and whether it is an acute episode or part of a chronic condition. Even if the clinical transaction is a one-off encounter, for example the patient is a temporary resident or the doctor a locum, it will often proceed smoothly and effectively. That this is so is, among other things, evidence of the regulatory influence of the social roles of doctor and patient.

Clearly many clinical transactions, as with Mrs Black, are straightforward. Sometimes, however, for a great variety of reasons, patients or doctors may depart from the constraints of their social roles. The scene is then set for such a departure, by one participant, to be amplified and perpetuated by an ill-advised or unwitting response from the other. An extreme example of this is when the patient and doctor become sexually involved. The patient has departed from normal illness behaviour and the doctor abandoned an appropriate professional stance. When this happens, the clinical transaction is no longer straightforward but has become complicated. Minor or transient departures from straightforward clinical transactions are common. Indeed these may be inevitable and, in fact, add zest and individuality to the particular doctor–patient interaction. Nor does the development of a complicated clinical transaction necessarily represent therapeutic failure, since it may be an unavoidable step in the progress to an ultimately satisfactory outcome (see Chapters 6 and 7). Clinical transactions are, therefore, of two main types – straightforward and complicated.

Straightforward clinical transactions

A straightforward clinical transaction is defined as: *a clinical transaction in which, as far as is appropriate, clinical goals are negotiated and a management strategy agreed that is conscientiously pursued by doctor and patient until a mutually acceptable termination (or agreement not to terminate) is achieved.*

The consultation between Mrs Black and her doctor is an example of a straightforward clinical transaction. Although termed straightforward, this type of clinical transaction demands that a number of preconditions are met and a number of stages successfully negotiated. These preconditions and stages can be teased out and enumerated (Table 2.1). Most clinical transactions probably do conform, overall, to the straightforward type, even if they digress temporarily along the way. However, every doctor will be familiar with clinical transactions that somehow become sidetracked and in which clear clinical goals are increasingly hard to

Table 2.1. *Pre-conditions or stages required of straightforward clinical transactions*

(1) The patient seeks appropriate health care based on
(2) an accurate self-perception of illness and/or symptoms and
(3) trusts in the doctor, which leads to
(4) a timely presentation to the doctor, who is
(5) suitably trained, and
(6) well-disposed towards the patient, and thus
(7) able to accurately diagnose any medical disorder and
(8) deliver the appropriate treatment[a], reassurance, information or explanation, leading to
(9) acceptance of the same by the patient, who
(10) within the expected time returns to a state of health or acceptable level of adjustment to any continuing illness

[a] Or referral to another more appropriate treatment resource.

identify or are lost sight of altogether. This situation may resolve itself as time goes on. Quite often, however, doctor and patient appear tacitly to agree to pursue a relationship that serves personal needs rather than particular clinical goals. Doctor and patient may become friends, and even deep attachments can develop, in the context of which clinical concerns are dealt with as almost incidental to the relationship. Even though a certain depth of relationship is necessary, especially when an extremely painful or distressing illness, or issues concerning terminal care, are involved, it should be borne in mind that any departure from the preconditions or stages in the straightforward clinical transaction can test the patient's or doctor's capacity to sustain their respective role responsibilities within the transaction. (Some of the factors that influence this capacity are considered in more detail in Chapter 4.)

The preconditions outlined above serve, therefore, as a baseline against which departures from the straightforward clinical transaction can be measured. Sometimes even minor departures can become amplified, driving the interaction to the point where the successful negotiation of a given stage in the transaction becomes arduous if not impossible.

Complicated clinical transactions

A complicated clinical transaction occurs when there is: *a significant, non-transitory, departure from the straightforward clinical transaction.*

Evidence for such departure may appear on either side of the doctor–patient interaction and at any stage in the transaction, which may span more than one consultation. The following clinical example serves to illustrate what is meant.

Mr Crown was a temporary resident and not registered with the family doctor involved. He was a large man with dark hair, and deeply tanned face and hands. He had a somewhat aggressive manner. He developed a sore throat, cough and fever and feeling generally unwell presented himself at reception and asked brusquely to see a doctor. He insisted on seeing a doctor that morning even though he was informed that there were no free appointments. As he stood close to the reception counter, his size and manner were experienced as intimidating by the receptionist, who agreed to see if he could be accommodated. The receptionist briefly told the doctor of Mr Crown's demands. The doctor, already behind in his schedule, grudgingly agreed to see Mr Crown. He decided that refusing to see him might have caused greater problems.

When Mr Crown was finally called he entered the consulting room and sat down. The doctor, somewhat taken aback by Mr Crown's great size, moved back in his chair. He asked unsmilingly what the problem was. Mr Crown detailed his symptoms and expressed his concern that he might have meningitis. He indicated he would like to be prescribed an antibiotic. Throughout, he sat very still, with a fixed and unblinking gaze. Without examining him, the doctor dismissed Mr Crown's concern about meningitis and told him that he was suffering from nothing more than a 'bad cold', which in fact required no treatment, other than simple symptomatic relief. Mr Crown was clearly unhappy with this diagnosis and advice and, leaning forward, he asserted that he always had antibiotics when he was 'like this' and would get much worse if he did not have them. Although reiterating that an antibiotic was really unnecessary, after further posturing on both sides, the doctor wrote out a prescription. Mr Crown scrutinised the prescription and declared that usually he had another brand of antibiotic. The doctor, by now feeling irritated, insisted that what he had prescribed would do perfectly well and Mr Crown, looking doubtful, left the room. Two days later he returned to the surgery and saw another doctor who prescribed the preferred antibiotic. Mr Crown was not seen again.

In terms of meeting the preconditions for a straightforward clinical transaction the above transaction can be seen to depart at a number of points, which will be looked at in turn. Although Mr Crown does indeed appear to seek appropriate health care, and his perception of his symptoms may be accurate, he regards them as more serious than does his doctor. The presentation may be timely but not so in terms of the doctor's appointment system! The question might be raised as to whether a 'bad cold' needs a doctor's advice at all. However, more important is the question of Mr Crown's trust in his doctor. There is little evidence of a trusting relationship but it is impossible to tell if this lack of trust applies to the particular doctor or to doctors in general. The doctor is apparently suitably trained and able to diagnose, although he refrains from a physical examination of the patient. From the outset, the doctor is not well disposed towards his patient. The advice and treatment given are contradictory and not accepted by Mr Crown, who returns for a second opinion.

Both the process and outcome of the clinical transaction between Mr Crown and his doctor indicate that this is a complicated transaction. The most significant departures from the preconditions of the straightforward transaction derive from personal factors, namely the trust of the patient and the attitude of the doctor. These complicating factors become amplified in their interaction and the outcome is unsatisfactory.

The stability of clinical transactions

The preconditions to be met, if a clinical transaction is to remain straightforward, place considerable demands on both patient and doctor. There is thus a pull towards complication, at least in certain interactions. This arises from any factor or collection of factors that compromise the carrying out of the reciprocal social roles of doctor and patient. The complication may begin in either the patient or the doctor or else in both simultaneously. Familial or wider social or personal aspects may influence the clinical transaction to be other than straightforward. Although personal factors such as friendliness and the capacity to empathise (see Chapter 4) can enhance the transaction, other factors can exert a powerful adverse effect. These tend to be negative attributes, for example envy, resentment or vengefulness, which under certain circumstances can emerge to influence the transaction. It is important to bear in mind, however, that strong positively toned emotions may also affect the transaction adversely (examples of this are discussed later). The inherent potential for powerful negative or positive factors to emerge unwittingly and unbidden during a transaction makes all clinical transactions intrinsically unstable and, as a consequence, liable to become complicated. There is a tension, therefore, between straightforward and complicated forms of the clinical transaction at any point in time and, paradoxically, the complicated clinical transaction is the more stable. This is because more is demanded of doctor and patient, in terms of psychological and social functioning, in maintaining a straightforward clinical transaction.

The effect of the illness itself may strain the patient's or doctor's capacity to maintain the straightforward transaction. Too little anxiety, for example, and patients may fail to seek help or present late; too much and they may present repeatedly with minor symptoms. Doctors, for their part, may feel anxious in the face of an illness or condition with which they are not familiar and therefore lacking in therapeutic confidence. In such a situation the response might be to minimise the gravity of the problem and failure to treat it adequately may be the result. Alternatively, the doctor might exaggerate the problem and overtreat or else refer inappropriately to a secondary care physician. The doctor may feel time-pressed or overtired. Under such circumstances the public level of the transaction may become complicated by a rushed history or physical examination that then leads to a missed or mistaken diagnosis. Too little time spent on explanation and instruction may make it harder for the patient to understand the illness and comply with treatment or advice. At the personal level, doctors may resent feeling time-pressed and, in effect blaming their patients for this, end up resenting them. Patients, sensing this, may feel offended, hurt, or resentful of their doctors' haste, inattention and apparent lack of concern.

As noted earlier, personal factors tend to arise inadvertently in the transaction and are consequently difficult to anticipate. A clinical transaction is all the more likely to become complicated if patient and doctor have been primed by previous transactions that have departed from the straightforward. In some circumstances difficulties can escalate to the point where there is a serious failure of the relationship as a whole. This may lead to patients being put off practice lists, complaints against doctors, or dangerous lapses of medical care. The following clinical example is an example of this last kind.

Mr Daniels, in his early forties, was not under normal circumstances a frequent attender at the surgery. He then visited several times within a short space of time complaining of a headache. His doctor, who hitherto had got on well with Mr Daniels, examined him carefully but, finding no signs of significant disease, sought to reassure him. Mr Daniels' visits continued, however, and his doctor came to regard him as overanxious, somatising the stress of a demanding occupation.

Mr Daniels did indeed have a stressful job and seemingly accepted his doctor's diagnosis, albeit reluctantly. He agreed to take a short course of a mild tranquilliser and to try to reduce the stress in his life and not to worry unduly about his physical symptoms. Some months elapsed before Mr Daniels attended again. He complained that his headaches were more severe and he had been vomiting. His doctor, not without showing some irritation, examined him again. This time, however, there was clear evidence of raised intracranial pressure and Mr Daniels was admitted to hospital. After a stormy course Mr Daniels recovered from a craniotomy to remove a large meningioma.

The overall clinical transaction in this case was complicated on both public and personal levels. The condition was not accurately diagnosed until it was almost too late. That this was so was due, in part, to the doctor's mounting impatience with Mr Daniels and the latter's response to this. Although nothing would have altered the ultimate diagnosis, or indeed the need for a craniotomy, appropriate treatment need not, perhaps, have been delayed to such a perilously late stage.

There are many clinical transactions, especially in primary care settings, often occurring in the context of a long and stable doctor–patient relationship, which seem superficially straightforward but are, in reality, complicated. As noted earlier, such transactions often serve some personal need of the doctor and patient as well as, or indeed in place of, the straightforward pursuit of clinical goals. Whereas this sort of relationship often has a positive value, this need not always be the case, as the example below demonstrates.

Mrs Evans was a regular and frequent attender at the surgery. At fifty-five, for a long time she had been unable to work because of severe, chronic asthma. In spite of this she continued to smoke several cigarettes per day. Despite its severity, her asthma was mostly stable. Her male doctor, considerably younger than her, regarded her as a warm individual and had an obvious liking for her. Their encounters involved making repeated minor alterations to her treatment, which never quite seemed to suit her, and mildly worded exhortations to stop smoking. Neither party ever engaged with the other in an open and appropriately serious or plain-speaking manner. What was never addressed by either, was the fact that, on occasion, Mrs Evans suffered acute exacerbations of her asthma that were truly life-threatening. These episodes almost always occurred when the doctor was away on holiday. It was as if both adopted a fatalistic view of Mrs Evans' illness without, however, being able to speak about it.

Complicated clinical transactions such as this, which are probably very common, may continue unrecognised. Clues to the complicated nature of the transaction may be subtle but can often be found if the doctor self-consciously examines feelings, thoughts, attitudes and behaviour stirred up in the interaction with the patient. In the case of Mrs Evans it was the absence of appropriate concern and a somewhat infantilising attitude that marked the deviation from the doctor's usual, rather business-like style. It took the doctor almost two years, however, before he recognised and acknowledged this to be the case (a trainee doctor sitting in with him remarked to this effect). In participating in the friendly but unchallenging relationship with Mrs Evans, the doctor came to realise that he was placing her life at greater risk.

Some clinical transactions, although not amounting to a separate type, reasonably tax the doctor's or patient's resources by virtue, for example, of the difficulty of the diagnostic task, in the case of an obscure masked or rare illness, or the discomfort, pain or other difficulty involved in the treatment. Difficulties in this context, include problems with communication due to learning disability, language, social or cultural barriers. Transactions that properly warrant secondary referral are often, although by no means always, likely to be complex. Nevertheless, in many instances, in spite of inherent complexities, the preconditions and stages of the straightforward clinical transaction are more or less stably met. However, complexity strains the transaction and such clinical transactions as a result run a higher risk of becoming complicated than do less-complex clinical transactions.

Three particular sets of factors strain the capacity of doctor and patient to maintain the straightforward transaction: (1) is the impact of the patient's complaint or illness itself; (2) adverse influences arising from the interaction of the individual personalities of patient and doctor; (3) complicating factors deriving from influences 'external' to the clinical transaction itself, as when duties concerning family or the workplace to which patient or doctor belong conflict with the goals of the clinical transaction (see Chapter 5). However, it is not possible to define any of these factors in isolation from the others, since they are all affected, and partly determined, by their interaction.

Many personal factors in the doctor–patient interaction are likely, under ordinary circumstances, to be operating outside of conscious awareness and are inescapable. Even the most straightforward of clinical transactions is also pursued at the personal level, which in most cases will be sufficiently robust to support the public level of the interaction and

make no difference to the overall straightforwardness of the transaction
and the securing of clinical goals. The doctor should approach the
transaction, however, with an understanding that the appropriate performance of the patient's role demands a considerable level of psychosocial
achievement that in some instances may exceed the patient's capacity.
After all, treatment might involve following complex protocols or require
a considerably amount of self-discipline if, for instance, lifestyle changes
are called for. Patients must, to some extent at least, also place themselves
trustingly in their doctors' hands, in the face of an illness they may only
poorly understand and the effects of which they may find very frightening.
This requires some capacity for mature dependence on the doctor, which
the patient may not have gained during his or her formative years (as
discussed in Chapter 3). Under such circumstances, the doctor may
have to cope with the emergence in the clinical transaction of seemingly
inappropriate and immature behaviour deriving from impoverished personal functioning (see Chapter 3). The situation will be aggravated if the
doctor, under the influence of aspects of his or her own personality,
automatically reacts to these or retaliates rather than taking them into
account.

Of course, the doctor's personal consultation style may, in fact, enhance
the likelihood of the transaction proceeding straightforwardly. But what
constitutes an appropriate consultation style, as was noted in Chapter 1,
is as difficult to define as what constitutes a problem patient. What is an
appropriate style will also tend to vary from patient to patient and from
stage to stage during a given clinical transaction. Good clinical communication skills, such as sufficient direct eye contact or the asking of
open and closed questions, as appropriate, may be learned to a degree
but they may be difficult to sustain if the patient's presentation arouses
powerful negative, or positive, emotions in the doctor or, more mundanely,
in the face of the doctor's boredom or fatigue.

The doctor has two sources of evidence that can be drawn on to decide
whether or not a clinical transaction has become complicated. On the
public level, a failure of compliance with, or delivery of, treatment or the
unexpected failure of the patient to recover (in the absence of misdiagnosis
or inappropriate treatment) indicates departure from the straightforward
transaction and may be obvious from the outset. Departures on the
personal level may be much more difficult to detect. Any noticeable,
non-transitory feelings or emotions that are not a familiar part of the
doctor's usual style of transacting should raise in his or her mind the
possibility of complication. It is important to remember, however, as is

emphasised elsewhere in this book, that personal level departures may be outside awareness and, paradoxically, surface only as departures from straightforward within the public domain. Thus, for example, a sensitive patient, offended by the doctor's brusque, albeit usual consultative style, may fail to comply with treatment. As far as the doctor is concerned the departure is on the public level, since the brusqueness, of which he or she is oblivious, does not indicate an ill-disposition toward the patient.

The transaction window

Having decided that a transaction has become complicated, or as a way of checking whether there have been any departures from the straightforward, doctors can organise information about the transaction by using a 'transaction window'. The transaction window is a simple four-celled diagrammatic representation of the clinical transaction defined by **Doctor, Patient, Public** and **Personal** (domains) as in Figure 2.1. It is constructed from the doctor's perspective. The doctor records the information about departures from the straightforward clinical transaction, using the preconditions of the straightforward transaction as a baseline within the four cells. The allocation of information into the different areas of the clinical transaction is illustrated in Figure 2.2. The window represents a snapshot of the clinical transaction and as such it cannot do justice to the ongoing process of the doctor–patient interaction. Thus, recognising in which domain a departure from the straightforward clinical transaction has arisen does not provide any information about the origins of the complication nor about how best the doctor might intervene.

Doctors' public domain responsibilities are that they should be suitably trained, able to diagnose and offer appropriate treatment, reassurance,

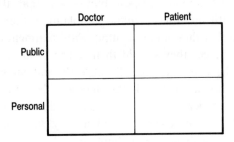

Figure 2.1. The transaction window.

	Doctor	Patient
Public	(5) Suitably trained (7) Able to accurately diagnose (8) Able to deliver appropriate treatment/advice/ explanation	(1) Patient seeks appropriate health care (2) Has an accurate self-perception of illness and/or symptoms (4) Timely presentation to doctor (9) Accepts treatment/advice and information (10) Returns to acceptable level of health
Personal	(6) Well-disposed toward patient	(3) Trusts doctor

Figure 2.2. The preconditions of the straightforward clinical transaction allocated to the four 'panes' of the transaction window.

advice and information or explanation. Departure from any of these preconditions complicates the transaction. Being suitably trained obiously means more than having completed medical training. In everyday clinical transactions doctors may be faced with situations at or beyond the limits of their competence. Common examples might be the undertaking of minor surgical procedures in primary care practice, without having had specific appropriate instruction, or taking on in-depth counselling or psychotherapy without the training and supervision necessary. In such instances, the risk is that the treatment will be inappropriate and the outcome unsuccessful or, at worst, damaging.

Patients' public domain responsibilities are that they should seek appropriate health care for a genuine complaint, in time for treatment to be effective and that they should comply with treatment or advice. Under normal circumstances they should then return to an acceptable level of health within the expected time. Because the patient may have health beliefs that do not accord with the doctor's, departures in the public domain of the clinical transaction may need mutual discussion and clarification. Doctors may need to explain why they are not able to deal with a particular problem and patients explain, for example, why they dispute the doctor's advice.

Using the transaction window

Monitoring the public level of the clinical transaction is a routine part of everyday clinical work and involves the continual re-evaluation of differential diagnosis and treatment. Monitoring of the personal level of the transaction, at least in a self-conscious way, is almost certainly less routinely carried out. The two requirements for the straightforward clinical transaction that lie most obviously in the personal domain are the doctor's disposition towards the patient and the patient's trust in the doctor. With some patients with diagnosable personality disorder, there may be little problem in detecting personal factors that might complicate the clinical transaction (see Appendix II). As emphasised earlier and illustrated by the case of Mr Daniels' meningioma, however, a small, unwitting departure from the well-disposed attitude, coupled with a failure of trust, can cause escalation to the point where the quality of the clinical work is jeopardised with attendant serious risks to patients' health. Attention should be paid, therefore, to any significant, non-transient distortions (thoughts, feelings, attitudes and behaviour) of the doctor's and patient's usual or conventional style of relating to one another.

The assumption is made here that patient and doctor are, in most clinical transactions, acting within the bounds of normal illness behaviour and a corresponding traditional professional stance. There are no doubt many instances of doctor–patient interaction that are habitually carried on in ways that stretch or breach these conventional boundaries. All doctors are likely to have relationships of this sort with at least a few of their patients. However, any clinical work undertaken in such doctor–patient interactions may suffer as a consequence. Motives for such relationships derive from personal factors that are often not conscious and therefore may be difficult to acknowledge and modify. Where significant clinical problems persistently arise because of such personal factors, this may be much more obvious to colleagues than to the relevant doctor. Exploring the reasons for complicated clinical transactions may, on this account, be more effectively done as a peer group exercise (see Chapter 8).

The transaction window creates four areas into which any evidence of complication, detected by monitoring the clinical transaction on public and personal levels, may be located. Departures from the straightforward may be seen to occur in the area of the doctor's or the patient's public domain activity; or they may be detected in the personal domain activity of patient or doctor. However, recognising a complication in one area does not imply that the cause of that complication lies in the same area or even within the same domain. This is because of the interactive effect (indicated by arrows between windows) whereby a departure in one domain can create a departure in the other and vice versa. Nor does locating a departure in one area indicate where any corrective intervention should be made. A departure identified in the public domain of the patient, for instance, may be best rectified by an altered personal aspect on the part of the doctor (see Chapters 6 and 7).

Dr Andrews noticed that one of his patients never complied with the treatment he advised, although he felt he gave clear and precise instructions. On discussion with colleagues, it was suggested that with this patient, Dr Andrews' rather gruff manner (which he himself saw as an expression of his cynical sense of humour) might be interpreted by the patient as dismissive and as authoritarian and thus be resented, and that non-compliance was the patient's way of responding to this. In the light of this, Dr Andrews agreed to modify his style with this patient and the improved relationship that followed seemed to lead to much better treatment compliance, supporting the original findings of the analysis of the transaction problem.

Transaction windows for this particular clinical situation might be created as shown in Figure 2.3. In this example, the initial complication was detected in routine public level monitoring within the area of the patient's public domain. The doctor's style was mooted as another possible complicating factor (although it should be noted that it was colleagues who supplied this entry to the transaction window) and it was speculated (hence in parentheses) that this caused resentment, i.e. was the hypothesised reason for poor compliance. An alteration in the doctor's personal domain had the desired result. Although apparently simple, this case entailed that the doctor both acknowledge that his personal style of consulting might be the cause of the problem and agree to modify it, at least experimentally for this particular patient.

Mr Adams, who suffered from congestive cardiac failure, persistently presented dangerously late with severe, acute exacerbations. The patient seemed nervous and suspicious of medical staff. The doctor allowed extra time to explain how the treatment ought to benefit the patient, in particular providing reassurance about possible side effects of his medication and emphasising the importance and advantage of early presentation in the acute phase. The patient was able to relax and appeared happy with this advice.

In this case complications were located in the patient's public domain behaviour and in his personal domain attitude. An intervention in the

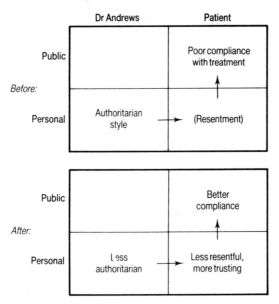

Figure 2.3. Transaction windows showing the interaction between Dr Andrews and his patient, before and after a change in consultation style. Arrows indicate the direction of hypothesised causal interaction and parentheses the patient's hypothesised personal aspect for which no direct or confirmed evidence was available at the time of discussion.

public domain, the delivery of appropriate reassurance, information and explanation from the doctor, led to a more trusting attitude in the patient and an expectation that this might lead to earlier presentation in future episodes. Transaction windows might be constructed as shown in Figure 2.4.

Working with transaction windows can become part of the doctor's everyday practice with every patient. It can readily become second nature, whether or not a window is literally constructed on each occasion. However, it can also be utilised in a small group setting, within a trusting and constructive atmosphere, as part of peer group supervision or between more senior supervising doctors and their juniors. This is, in part, because it is relatively easy to locate complications in the public domain or in the patient's personal domain (hence the 'problem patient') but not so easy for doctors to objectively evaluate their own personal contributions to complicated transactions. Audiotape or videotape recordings can obviously be of great value (see Chapter 9).

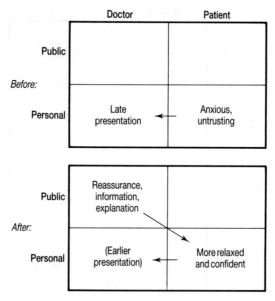

Figure 2.4. Transaction windows indicating the effect of the doctor's reassurance (public domain intervention) on Mr Adams. Parentheses indicate hypothesised or expected change.

A source of complication in clinical transactions may derive from a conflict between the goals of the clinical transaction, as a system, and the goals of other systems to which doctor or patient may separately and simultaneously belong. In a primary care setting, for example, not uncommonly a doctor might want to finish evening surgery in good time because of family or social commitment. The last patient poses a difficult clinical management problem that will take some time to sort out. Being a member of both the clinical transaction and the family system the doctor has to manage conflicting demands on his or her time. Such a conflict can increase the risk of a complicated transaction – if not in the surgery, then at home! Such an example is familiar to most doctors. In less obvious cases it can be of value to construct a window for the transaction that overlaps with the clinical transaction (Figure 2.5; see also Chapter 5).

In Figure 2.5 the broken arrows indicate where a complicating effect may impact on the patient. A transaction window is included for an overlapping patient system should this be relevant. With familiarity, windows can be rapidly sketched and left unlabelled, and arrows indicating

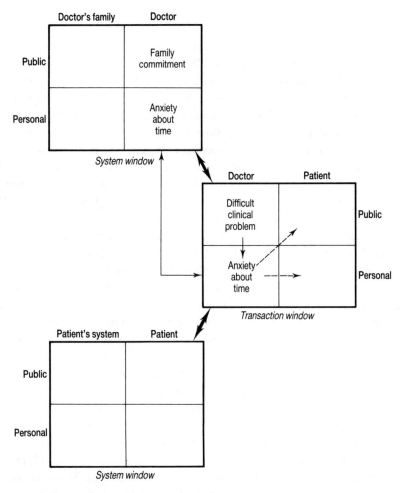

Figure 2.5. Transaction windows indicating the influence of aspects of the doctor's family system on the clinical transaction. The patient's family system may also influence the clinical transaction.

important interactions quickly drawn. In a tutorial session between trainer and trainee doctor, for example, it may be sufficient just to have empty windows, drawing in the arrows and simply talking about the content of the individual window panes, once the departure from the straightforward clinical transaction has been identified and placed in the relevant square. Further examples are given in later chapters.

Conclusions

There are two main types of clinical transaction – straightforward and complicated. Either form is potentially present at any given point during the clinical encounter. The two forms of the transaction exist as if in dynamic tension with one another. Because performing the respective roles of doctor and patient may demand more of either participant than they are capable of, the straightforward clinical transaction is the less stable. It is especially liable to become complicated under the influence of personal aspects of the doctor–patient interaction. Such personal factors are often inadvertent, outside awareness and subtle. Any non-transient and significant departures from the straightforward clinical transaction indicate the development of a complicated clinical transaction.

The transaction window provides a diagrammatic representation of the clinical transaction, at a single point in time. It divides the transaction into four areas in which the complicating departure(s) can be located. These are the doctor's public domain activity, the patient's public domain activity and the personal domains of doctor and patient. On account of the interactive effect of doctor on patient and public on personal domain (and vice versa), locating a complication in one area does not indicate in which area the cause, or indeed the solution, is to be found. Even so, the transaction window serves as a convenient shorthand or summary of the nature of the clinical transaction, yielding a visible statement of any departures from the straightforward. It also provides a format for hypothesising the site and likely effect of therapeutic interventions. An additional strength of this analytical approach to clinical transactions resides in the interactive aspect, i.e. that trainer and trainee or colleagues use the transaction window as an active analytical tool. Thus, working with transaction windows is usefully undertaken in groups, as well as part of solitary practice, especially in order to obtain a more objective view of personal domain material, such as aspects of a doctor's personal style. To evaluate the potentially complicating influence of contextual factors, a system window can also prove valuable.

3

Interpersonal influences

Introduction

Ms King suffered from diabetes mellitus that was hard to stabilise, partly on account of her poor compliance with medication and partly due to her failure to curb her craving for chocolate. She would begin a consultation in a rather timid and self-deprecating manner. However, with little or no warning she would move from this childlike posture into a verbally abusive tirade against the doctor whenever he, no matter how tactfully, tried to indicate that she had a part to play in the suboptimal management of her condition. The doctor believed that he was experienced as somebody who was entirely uncaring. Since his view of himself was very different from this, he found himself rising to the bait of her provocation and reacting with annoyance. He thus tended, at least from time to time, to enter into active confrontation and direct criticism of the patient. In effect, he was turned into somebody who indeed appeared uncaring. The result was a kind of instability within the doctor–patient relationship that was inadequate to support the successful pursuit of the clinical goal of stabilising the diabetes.

Clinical transactions may become complicated for a variety of reasons and evidence for the complication may surface, to be recognised as such, within either public or personal (if not both) levels of the doctor–patient interaction. Evidence for departure from the straightforward clinical transaction, within the public domain, is often obvious, since it may involve gross, behavioural departure, for example poor compliance with treatment as with Ms King. Consequently, it may be discovered before other departures, which may be more subtle, although no less significant in terms of their complicating effect. The clinical transaction, therefore, may be complicated long before it is recognised by the doctor to be so, especially when initially the only actual evidence is within the personal domain and also of a subtle kind. Potentially, departures are the more powerful in their distortion of the clinical transaction the longer they remain covert. This point cannot be emphasised too much.

The goals of the public domain are synonymous with the clinical goals that relate to the interaction of doctor and patient as they perform their respective social roles. Those of the personal domain refer to the maintaining of the necessary quality of the interaction and are more relevant to process than to any particular clinical goal. The implicit general goal of the personal level of interaction, however, is to provide a sufficiently trusting and confiding relationship, within which the business of achieving clinical goals can be carried on. Of course the public and personal domains interact (see Figure 3.1) and they can only be separated artificially.

Although the respective goals of the public and personal domains differ, they are not necessarily contradictory. However, sometimes this may be the case, for example, when a patient becomes overly dependent on the doctor, perhaps presenting repeatedly with minor or trivial symptoms as a means of maintaining inappropriate emotional dependence. The public level goal, in such an instance, might be to reduce dependency and yet the personal level goal requires a relationship, in which such dependency issues may be explored. Paradoxically, the doctor is in the position of fostering a relationship with the ultimate goal of its rupturing or, at least, its being carried on within defined limits.

To monitor the success of the clinical transaction represents a simpler task within the public domain. Within the personal domain, monitoring is made difficult because: (1) such signs are not customarily discussed openly by doctor and patient, nor are related to explicit goals; (2) they

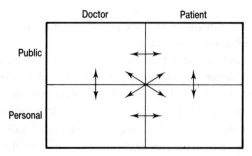

Figure 3.1. The transaction window with arrows indicating that factors in all areas of the window may interact.

arise from the personal interaction of doctor and patient as people (i.e. not simply as players of their respective roles); (3) they derive from unconscious factors attributes, otherwise appearing to happen automatically or spontaneously, without conscious thought or planning; and (4) some signs of departure are subtle.

Particularly when the clinical transaction is complex (see p. 27), the doctor will already have many other aspects to attend to and, as a result, less mental space, time and energy available for monitoring the personal domain. Neglect of personal domain monitoring, however, can allow the development of significant departures from the straightforward clinical transaction. Through the effect of such departures on the process of the interaction, the outcome too can be adversely affected.

Psychodynamic perspective

A psychodynamic perspective can shed light on the shifting, dynamic nature of the personal interaction between doctor and patient, as they engage in the process of negotiating and securing the relevant clinical goals. Such a perspective allows for an understanding of the reasons for, and mechanisms of, the departure from the straightforward clinical transaction through an analysis of, on the one hand, the maintaining of a well-disposed attitude and consultation style of the doctor, and, on the other hand, the capacity of the patient to trust, confide in and appropriately depend upon the doctor. In particular, a psychodynamic perspective permits an examination of unconscious motivation (and goals) of both doctor and patient, the influence of the personality of doctor and patient in their interaction, and the influence of their past relationships with significant others (most notably parents and other authority figures) on the current style and quality of relating and interacting.

A psychodynamic perspective is directly relevant to the personal interaction and only indirectly so to the public level. Its use, as a conceptual tool, complements the sociological (especially, social role theory) and systemic approaches (see Chapters 1 and 5). It represents an in-depth method of examination that goes beyond the understanding available from an application of the other two conceptual approaches. However, all three models are required for a comprehensive understanding of clinical transactions and they can be applied together.

In this chapter personality development and unconscious motivation are discussed from a psychodynamic perspective, highlighting their relevance to clinical transactions. The influence of past relationships on current psychological and social functioning is examined in Chapter 4.

Personality development

The origins of personality development remain obscure. Genetic and environmental factors combine in their effect and neither can be clearly disentangled. This having been said, most individuals with abnormal personalities, hence certain patients who come into contact with doctors, have histories that betray important early environmental influences of an adverse kind. The fact of this history is often obscured, however, by the patient's overt display of attitudes and behaviour, a façade that masks underlying frailty or vulnerability and may, as a consequence, serve to deflect the doctor's attention from it. Thus, some of the most psychologically damaged personalities present, in certain situations and under particular circumstances, in an apparently happy, confident or even aggressive manner that may serve to discourage the doctor from eliciting a history that might document early emotional deprivation or abusive experiences.

Mr Johns appeared as a lively and bright single man in his early thirties when he presented to his new family doctor, having recently moved into a rented flat in the area. Previous case records were unavailable and the only information was that elicited at this first consultation. Mr Johns revealed a history of serious gastroenterological problems for which he had undergone extensive surgery and required long-term medication, the empty bottles for which he produced as evidence. Mr Johns' new doctor found Mr Johns to be a truly remarkable character who had endured his chronic illness and attendant complications with great fortitude. What especially impressed the doctor was Mr Johns' apparent acceptance of his state of ill health and his respect, humility and gratitude to the medical profession. The doctor did wonder, as Mr Johns left the consultation with effusive thanks for the repeated prescription of tablets, that there might be a degree of obsequiousness in Mr Johns' manner, but in spite of this (which he chided himself had been an uncharitable thought under the circumstances) he retained an extremely favourable impression, noting that he had felt almost moved to tears by the encounter.

Mr Johns' doctor was surprised to read from the case-notes, when they arrived a week later, that Mr Johns had served several terms of imprisonment for aggravated burglary and also had a lengthy history of alcohol and multiple drug misuse. Reading the notes, with a degree of incredulity, he discovered that Mr Johns had experienced an extremely chaotic early life, with mother taking many partners and the family making many moves of house that severely interrupted his schooling and peer relationships. Mr Johns had been physically abused by two of his 'stepfathers', one of whom also sexually abused him. It was noted, however, that Mr Johns was a charming and personable man.

Another example of adverse early circumstances that may be masked or not elicited is that of battering parents who themselves in childhood were victims of physical abuse. In part, the situation may be understood as individuals, internalising, through learning and experiencing, not only their own part in the interaction with authority figures (especially parents) but also that of the authority figures themselves. In the case of a child victim of physical abuse, therefore, what is internalised is something of the whole abuser–abused relationship, i.e. not only the experience of being a victim but also, vicariously, something of that of the victimiser. Thus, later in life, both internalised aspects (victim and victimiser) are potentially available for re-experiencing and re-enacting, according to the circumstances. Such adult individuals may be objectively identifiable as victimisers, while their own sense of themselves may still be that of victims. At a given point in time, such an individual may be consciously identified with only one pole of the victim–victimiser psychodynamic theme, which characterises many, if not all, of their relationships. In many instances because of the damaging effect upon personality development of abuse or neglect in childhood there may be a poorly established sense of self and conscious motivation and, as a result, confusion between self and other, victim and victimiser.

Clearly the majority of infants, children and adolescents are not grossly abused, deprived or otherwise maltreated. However, the experience of being alive is intrinsically frustrating, since no individual's needs are ever perfectly met. As a result, part of human development involves acquiring strategies with which to deal with the inevitable frustrations and resultant psychic pain or anxiety of daily living. Early in development, strategies are unconsciously deployed, if for no other reason than that the infant's cognitive apparatus, hence ability to make conscious decisions, is immature. Also the individual's capacity to take action, in response to frustration, is curtailed. (Clearly emotional, intellectual and physical development carry on simultaneously but not necessarily hand in hand.) Thus, a given frustration at one stage of personality development may be less traumatic in its effect than if it occurs at a later stage. The cognitive apparatus (and body) may by then be more fully developed and able to cope via an enhanced ability to understand and hence potentially tolerate, and, if necessary, to take action in response to a particular frustration. Too much frustration, privation or insult, or too soon, means that the developing individual's resources are taxed and overwhelmed. Evidence of this will also differ according to the developmental stage and be under the influence of earlier stages and any associated difficulties. When excessive frustration or insult is repeated and habitual, extreme strategies, with which to attempt to cope with them, also become habitual. Therefore, with the passage of time, such aspects become part of the enduring characteristics of the functioning and organisation of an individual's personality. Their continuing presence is reinforced by the environmental response, which in part becomes shaped by aspects of the personality of the individual, for instance, choice of friends or partners.

The early developmental experience of children, therefore, critically affects the quality of the relationships they are capable of making with others, probably throughout the rest of their lives. Care-seeking and care-giving are intrinsic and reciprocal aspects of human social activity. They reflect part of the human need to form emotional attachments to others, over and beyond the need for food and sex (Bowlby, 1958). Repeated observation has shown that children develop distinguishable patterns of attachment in response to the ways in which they are treated by their carers (Ainsworth *et al.*, 1978; Main *et al.*, 1985). A particular pattern of attachment, once established as a working model of the self with resultant expectations of other people, has predictive value for the quality of future relationships. A child who, in adverse conditions, has had a sufficiently reliable response and helpful attention from loving parents is likely to develop a secure pattern of attachment. This goes hand in hand with the capacity to separate and explore the world, and to seek help, reassurance or comfort openly and trustingly. Children who have no such confidence in the availability, reliability and responsiveness of their care-givers are likely to become anxiously attached – fearful of separation and lacking in trust. If carried into adulthood, such patterns of behaviour will profoundly affect the capacity to both give and seek help or care, with obvious implications for the doctor–patient relationship.

Psychological defence mechanisms

The unconscious strategies of the mind, which protect against the adverse effect of too much frustration or anxiety, are termed psychological mechanisms of defence. The more the dose of frustration lies within the individual's capacity to deal with it, the less extreme will be the defence mechanisms employed. The function of any defence mechanism is to modulate the direct experience of the frustration. Thus, ultimately, the effect of a defence mechanism is to distort an accurate conscious perception of the reality of the frustrating situation. The more the mismatch between the extent of frustration and the individual's capacity to withstand it, the more the defence mechanism(s) deployed are required to distort the real situation. Defence mechanisms habitually deployed become part of the individual's characteristic or personal style of being and relating to others. When such extreme, and necessarily reality-distorting, strategies are habitually deployed, they become incorporated into the developing personality and thereby influence the subsequent development of the personality. In adulthood, therefore, an abnormal personality may be the result.

An abnormal personality may be marked by the absence or presence of various traits or characteristics depending, to some extent, on the precise details of the genetic endowment, environmental influences and coping strategies employed to deal with the combined effect of the genetic and environmental influences. When sufficiently severe, abnormality of the personality is referred to as being disordered. Personality disorder, a diagnostic term (see Appendix II), refers to significant suffering experienced, by virtue of the personality, or to a personality that brings about significant suffering to others or to society in general.

The relevance of a discussion of individuals' patterns of attachment and psychological defence mechanisms, in this context, is the particular effect certain of them exert in relationship to other people with whom they come into personal or professional contact. Also, certain defence mechanisms, acquired in response to particularly adverse circumstances during an individual's formative years, tend to cluster and be deployed in a relatively fixed, inflexible way that brings characteristic patterns of interactive style (Kernberg, 1975; Vaillant, 1992), especially within the context of an intimate or infantile dependent relationship, such as may exist between doctor and patient. The individuals concerned tend to become involved in interactive styles that are counter to direct communication with others and that confer a narrow repertoire of behavioural expressions and responses and hence constrain the interaction (such behaviour is more likely in those who have developed anxious as opposed to secure attachments in childhood). As a result, any interpersonal transactions in which such individuals are involved readily become complicated.

Maintaining an empathic relationship with them is also made more difficult. Clinical transactions involving such individuals will carry an increased likelihood of becoming complicated because of the reciprocal relationship of care-seeking and care-giving.

Ms Shah presented with constipation. She appeared happy to comply with answering questions about her bowel habit but became abruptly fearful when her doctor asked to physically examine her. With sympathetic questioning the doctor ascertained that Ms Shah had been severely sexually abused, including anal penetration. Consequently, the doctor concluded that it was fears stirred by memories of the abuse that prevented further investigation of the problem. Although feeling uneasy about prescribing medication for symptomatic relief without having carried out a physical examination, the doctor prescribed a laxative.

The doctor had also offered to refer Ms Shah to a female colleague but this offer had been declined. The doctor was surprised that Ms Shah had not taken up the offer but decided to offer regular weekly sessions of half an hour, in order to permit her to ventilate some of her fears regarding physical contact and abuse in the hope that this would desensitise her to being examined by him.

Ms Shah returned after two weeks with the problem unresolved and symptoms continuing. She accepted the offer of weekly sessions. However, the doctor soon realised that it was difficult to maintain a focus on issues to do with physical contact and abuse. Instead, Ms Shah would introduce, almost apologetically, a further symptom. For example, she revealed that she had self-induced vomiting. The doctor felt that this was a significant and potentially relevant symptom and he elicited a history of longstanding body image problems and associated eating disorder (bulimia nervosa). However, he became increasingly frustrated that no matter what the presented complaint the clinical transaction did not reach a satisfactory conclusion. Ms Shah, he believed, seemed to think that she could only maintain his interest by presenting a new symptom, of which she seemed to have a very large supply.

The presented symptoms did have the effect of engaging the doctor's professional curiosity and personal sympathy, at least during the first few weekly sessions. However, as time went on the doctor's own sense of frustration and impotence mounted as he realised he was unable to successfully tackle any of the presented problems. He lost his initial empathy with Ms Shah and became increasingly inwardly hostile in attitude toward her. He felt as though she were consciously thwarting his best attempts to help her and that even if she were to present the most eminently treatable and minor condition he would fail in his attempt to help her.

Conscious and unconscious motivation

Potential medical students are often asked, at interview for a place at medical school, what motivates them to become doctors. Obviously their answers vary. However, successful interviewees, as they subsequently pursue a career in the medical profession, may be aware of insights into their own motivation, which develop only with time and experience. This does not necessarily imply that motivation differs at subsequent stages in doctors' development, although this may be the case. It may be that, with the passage of time, original aspects of motivation become clearer. Earlier, motivation may thus have been present, although unconscious.

Likewise, the development of relationships, between individuals or the choice of friends or sexual partners, involves motivation that may not be entirely conscious. If asked to provide reasons for liking or loving a partner, a person may appear 'lost for words'. With time or prompting, he or she may be able to offer some insights but often, perhaps embarrassingly, there will appear to be insufficient justifications. Much of the motivational force, and argument, is not directly accessible to conscious scrutiny by the mind.

When it comes to the doctor–patient relationship and clinical transactions, therefore, there will be aspects of the personal interaction that appear merely to happen, without will or desire. For example, no deliberate act of will is experienced as being deployed in smiling a greeting to a familiar attractive patient. However, some personal aspects of the relationship, while not usually reflected upon and seldom discussed, may nevertheless be available for introspective examination (i.e. they are conscious). An example might be a degree of sexual attraction between doctor and patient. In most circumstances, a spoken acknowledgement of this is not required or appropriate. Doctor and patient will go about their respective social role activities, within the clinical transaction, and complete their business without prolonging or disturbing it by developing a sexual liaison.

Sometimes, however, aspects of the doctor–patient interaction are unconscious and therefore not accessible to introspection. As a result, such unconscious factors can affect the process of the clinical transaction, through an effect on the personal interaction, which may then impact upon the public domain and affect the securing of clinical goals. The task confronting the doctor, in attempting to monitor the personal level of the interaction, includes learning to recognise evidence of unconscious motives that may subvert or undermine the clinical transaction. The following clinical example may shed some light on this important issue.

A doctor became aware that a complicated clinical transaction was present only after her receptionist commented that she had noticed that Mrs Francis, who suffered from chronic rheumatoid arthritis, always received more than her allotted appointment time. The doctor considered the content of the consultations otherwise unremarkable. Having thought about the receptionist's observation, the doctor decided to attempt to keep within the normal time allocation (and usually she was quite strict about her time-keeping). Only then was she aware that her patient was extremely demanding, presenting myriad other complaints (not all of which were strictly medical) and also passively aggressive in manner. Recognising this, she was able, some time later, to make psychosocial enquiries (see Chapter 6), which revealed long-standing social phobic symptoms. These markedly curtailed Mrs Francis' social function. The patient had felt foolish and ashamed to have such difficulties and frustrated by her own inability to talk about her problems even with her doctor.

In this example, the public level of the doctor–patient interaction departed from the straightforward but the doctor had been oblivious to this until the receptionist made her observation. The doctor then construed the situation as the result of an unconscious communication at the personal level of her interaction with her patient, the effect of which was to make terminating the consultation difficult. She came to realise that she felt guilty, when bringing the consultation to a close, sensing that termination was experienced by Mrs Francis as rejection. Only when the doctor attempted to keep to the time boundaries of the appointment did the patient's negative feelings surface. It was only once she had ventilated her feelings that she was able to reveal her symptoms. The doctor recognised, however, that she herself had felt as if she needed to keep this patient happy at all costs (Figure 3.2). Perhaps, unconsciously, the doctor had feared entering into an angry exchange with her.

Albeit transiently, an angry and resentful patient did emerge and, indeed, the doctor did feel very uncomfortable during this phase but, largely, she retained her outward composure, resisting the temptation to

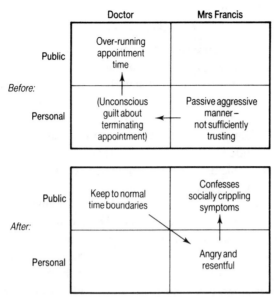

Figure 3.2. Transaction windows showing the interaction between the doctor and Mrs Francis, before and after the doctor's public domain intervention of keeping the consultation within normal time boundaries.

become too defensive. Seeing that the doctor accommodated her ventilation of frustration, the patient was able to confess her symptoms the more fully and, as a result, experienced considerable relief. After further examination of the extent of her psychosocial difficulties, the doctor referred her for behavioural treatment to a clinical psychologist, without the patient feeling rejected by her doctor.

The subtle departure from the straightforward clinical transaction, in the personal domain, was thus the doctor's unconscious wish to maintain a 'happy' relationship with her patient and her unconscious fear that an angry exchange would ensue to disrupt the relationship. The initial evidence for the departure was, in fact, within the public domain but the doctor was oblivious to this, i.e. unconscious of it. The public domain departure was fuelled by the unconscious fears and wishes within the personal domain. The combined influence was such that both doctor and patient were prevented from confronting their legitimate clinical concern, in this instance the crippling social phobia.

Complicating factors

Individuals who experience sufficient satisfying responses in their formative
years (implying an empathic or 'concordant' relationship with early
care-givers) come to experience themselves as essentially good people
inhabiting a relatively benign world (i.e. one that is sensitive and
responsive to their needs and demands) compared to those whose infantile
and later experiences have been predominantly frustrating. The former
establish an attitude of basic trust, rather than mistrust, secure as opposed
to anxious attachments and the beginnings of a capacity to depend
maturely upon other people.

At early stages of development, however, all infants will tend to
experience the same care-giver differently according to the dominant
affect, or feeling state, which operates during a given encounter. (The
residues of this situation exist with a potential for reactivation in
everybody.) Thus according to psychodynamic theory, the infant who is
frustrated by mother, experiences her as a 'bad' mother and vice versa,
i.e. as a 'good' mother when needs are being satisfied. It is only later, with
increased cognitive development, *together with* sufficient satisfactory
experiences, that a capacity develops that allows recognition of the fact
that the 'good' and 'bad' care-givers are aspects of the same individual
and this also allows the distinguishing of self from the other. Other people
are then experienced as distinct persons in their own right. However, the
capacity to tolerate and integrate ambivalence, love and hate, is not a
once-and-for-all phenomenon. Thus, the experiencing of the frustrating
other (for example, the doctor who fails to cure or the patient who fails
to recover) as an 'all bad' person may readily surface.

One important effect of the deployment of primitive and profoundly
reality-distorting mechanisms (reminiscent of those deployed in infancy
and in relation to repeated privation, frustration or abuse) is that the
other person in the relationship, in this instance the doctor or patient, is
experienced in contradictory ways. Thus, they may be experienced as
'good' (accepting or benevolent) at one time and, at another time, perhaps
only seconds later, as 'bad' (rejecting or malevolent). Another important
effect is that this same antithetic stance is applied to their experience of
the self. Thus, the individual's self-experience may also rapidly and
markedly fluctuate between extremes of goodness and potency on the
one hand and worthlessness and hopeless impotence on the other. In
certain individuals, fluctuations, as described above, are rapid and urgent
in their expression and in their effect on others. Too easily the potential

internal conflict of the patient (in attempting to resolve his or her conflicting aspects) become enacted interpersonally between patient and doctor.

Faced with this kind of presentation of extreme emotional and behavioural fluctuation in a patient (as in the case of Ms King and her unstable diabetes, quoted at the beginning of this chapter) the doctor may be bewildered and so may feel powerless about how best to respond and maintain professional composure. Very quickly, under such circumstances, there is a risk of frustration and impotence that may generate an expression of irritation or anger. This may be suppressed but, too easily, it can impact on the patient, if evidence of it is detected, and the effect can be to produce an angry stalemate from which the legitimate medical work is increasingly excluded.

Stalemate can be prolonged, since the patient's rapidly fluctuating and contradictory views of the doctor are, as it were, amplified by the doctor who, in effect, enacts the complementary pole of the patient's dominant psychodynamic theme, in the above example the uncaring and critical aspects. In the process the patient enacts the obverse of this. Thus, the patient, in this example, experiences herself as the person who is being wronged. Low self-worth in the patient is then exchanged (via the unconscious deployment of defence mechanisms) for a rather grandiose and offended self – the martyr – maligned and misunderstood. Through this the patient experiences temporary relief from her usual low self-esteem.

A doctor may resist the temptation to react out of frustration and sense the patient's pain at feeling ill used. This may then be meaningfully conveyed to, and accepted by, the patient and the stalemate may be broken (Figure 3.3). However, the enactment of personal aspects can leave, in its wake, difficulties that surface later and impair the quality of subsequent clinical transactions thereby increasing the risk of their becoming complicated. To some extent, any later negative impact can be avoided by discussing the situation that has taken place and by identifying some of the mechanisms and other factors involved. Ideally, however, familiarity with monitoring the personal level of interaction means that signs are detected early and the doctor can be alert to the risk of a complicated clinical transaction developing and take any necessary steps to preserve the straightforward form (see Chapters 6 and 7).

Patients who habitually deploy primitive and profoundly reality-distorting defence mechanisms have a chronically impaired sense of self, both in terms of their estimation of their own self-worth (which tends to

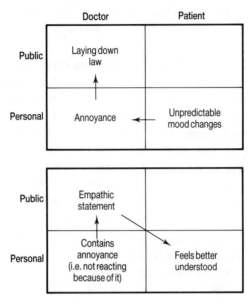

Figure 3.3. Transaction windows indicating how an empathic statement by the doctor might have broken the stalemate in the doctor's interaction with Ms King.

veer between extremes) and in terms of their capacity to differentiate themselves (ownership of attitudes, emotions and motives) from another person with whom they interact. In relation to an authority figure, or other situation that might generate anxiety, patients' capacities to distinguish what is their own self and what is the other's is markedly impaired. Thus it may be that instead of recognising their own hostility in the face of hearing about an unfavourable prognosis or unpalatable treatment, they experience hostility as a part of, and coming from, the person of the doctor. A simple example is the patient who, on hearing bad news regarding diagnosis, acts as if to hold the doctor responsible for this – accurate reality testing having given way to a persecutory mode of mental functioning. It is easy to imagine how any clinical transaction can be hampered by such an occurrence that happens regularly and not only in response to objectively serious matters.

In an attempt to compensate for, or adjust to, such long-term personal difficulties, the patient may have a social network including a family system, that acts to mask or else preserve a low self-esteem. Alternatively, the network might act to reinforce the intrinsically ambivalent elements within its relationships. To some extent, career or job choice may reflect aspects which can compensate for low self-esteem. Thus, if available, a job may be selected that masks a frail self-esteem by superimposing, via professional training, a public role that carries with it responsibility incorporating high status and power. Job choice of this sort does not necessarily reflect conscious motivation or choice (see above). Obviously even slight changes in the psychosocial support systems of such patients and doctors may have a powerful, and seemingly inappropriately large, effect on the consequent level of functioning. (Chapter 5 addresses the issue of the doctor and patient in their respective social systems and also the way in which such systems may interact.)

It may be that certain doctors have chosen their profession, at least in part, for unconscious motives such as just described. In as much as this is the case (and it should be noted that the phenomenon is not 'all or nothing'), the clinical transaction can be influenced in more or less predictable ways, because of this constellation of defensive manoeuvres within the doctor. Therefore, it may be that, as long as the patient is dependent, passive and submissive in attitude to the doctor or is a grateful patient (serving to boost the doctor's self-esteem) this meets the doctor's needs, and is indeed what by virtue of his or her professional role is expected. Once this is not the case, however, the scene is set for a complicated clinical transaction.

Conclusions

A psychodynamic perspective sheds light on the personal level of inter-action between doctor and patient. It is required because of the dynamic nature of human relationships, in which emotional responses and attitudes, both toward oneself and others, may fluctuate, sometimes at great speed. Fluctuation may be from one extreme to the other, as well as by degree. Also, it may bear little or no direct relation to what is going on in the public level of the interaction. Because of the possibility of extreme fluctuation and fluctuation at rapid pace, awareness of these phenomena is required, if a doctor is to avoid or minimise bewilderment and conse-quent frustration, the effect of which, through interaction with the public level interaction, will be to complicate the overall clinical transaction.

Certain individuals, whether doctors or patients, are more likely to become involved in complicated clinical transactions, generated via the route of an altered personal level of interaction. Those most at risk display the trademarks of primitive and profoundly reality-distorting psycho-logical defence mechanisms, which in the course of defending the mind of the individual by regulating the emotional effects of conflict or frustration, also exert an effect on others, especially those who are engaged within an intimate, infantile dependent or stressful contact (such as often pertains in the doctor–patient relationship). One common effect is to avoid the establishment of an empathic relationship. Those who have experienced abuse, deprivation or neglect in their formative years often have difficulty facing the prospect of intimate disclosure (because of an earlier experience of failure in trust and respect) and even asking for help or care for genuine and serious illness becomes problematic. This reflects an impoverished capacity to regulate self-esteem and difficulty differentiating their own from others' attitudes, feelings and motives.

The contribution of the human environment to the development of the adult personality is incorporated into the structure of the personality via combined 'self-other' memories and images, together with the emotional tone prevailing at the time, which create a characteristic working model of the self. Thus, in children this reflects the patterns of attachment formed with their carers. Current enduring relationships therefore have a style and emotional tone representing characteristics of the personality derived from earlier stages in its development, to which the individual will have more or less conscious access later. The more satisfactory and non-traumatising the earlier relationships (with parents or other usual care-givers) the less will be the use of the profoundly reality-distorting defences. These are not required so much because the level of anxiety or frustration is more or less consonant with the developing individual's capacity to tolerate or master these. Together with this, less reality-distorting defences can develop and these can be deployed, albeit also unconsciously, to equip the individual with a wider range of potential responses to novel or known frustrating situations and in relationship to other people. Such individuals are likely to have formed secure attachments as infants. They (largely but not entirely) avoid both the profoundly reality-distorting defence mechanisms and also the associated rigidity and fixity of their defensive styles, at least in the face of life's ordinary challenges. This enables them to respond appropriately to a range of individuals, according to the context, without becoming unduly mistrustful and thus they can transact with many different individuals and make reasonable and appropriate demands on others.

When defences are primitive and fixed, this often reflects the habitual experience of narrow, restrictive or emotionally and physically traumatising relationship styles. Rather than having, therefore, a range of styles of relating to others they tend to have a smaller repertoire based on certain dominant psychodynamic themes, sometimes only a single theme, for example, victim–victimiser, in which the individual appears to be only ever one or other extreme in relation to other people. Clearly, negotiation of clinical goals requiring compromise or compliance or active participation in treatment will be hampered under such conditions. A personality with such a restricted range of relationship styles tends to oscillate, sometimes quickly and dramatically, between the extremes and has little or no capacity to temper a response or find middle ground. This style of relating (which applies both to the relationship with the self as well as to others) has an effect on others with whom he or she comes into contact and is, in that sense, contagious.

Contagion happens partly because of the difficulty of the more mature personality in tolerating the empathic gymnastics required in order to keep pace with the less mature personality's posturing and contortions. As a result, the mature personality's less mature aspects are caused to resonate. The effect is to relieve the more immature personality of inner tension, previously generated by the non-integration of the contradictory and ambivalent attitudes to self and others. The immature personality thus becomes identified with only one psychodynamic pole (for example, victim) while the other person enacts the counterpart (the victimiser). Such a development may be surprisingly stable, as if fulfilling some unconscious needs of both participants. The more mature personality's attempts to shift the situation are often unsuccessful, generating further frustration, which increases the stress on that personality, thereby increasing the likelihood of more primitive functioning seemingly irrespective of the context.

4

The influence of past relationships

Introduction

Henry, an adolescent male, became a frequent presenter at surgery, requesting sick certification for depressed mood and self-mutilation. A full syndrome of depressive disorder, which might have justified a course of antidepressant medication, was never present. In any case, the patient had volunteered that he would 'never touch any drugs'. The self-mutilation was not serious enough to warrant medical treatment in its own right. The patient refused the doctor's invitation to discuss his psychosocial circumstances yet repeatedly returned to the surgery.

The three doctors in the primary care practice were equally irritated and frustrated by the patient's behaviour and resolved to confront him with their views of the unsatisfactory nature of the consultations. When this took place, an ugly scene ensued, in which Henry, who had taken alcohol, became physically threatening and eventually the police were called to remove him from the premises. The woman doctor who had confronted Henry had herself felt extremely aggressive and near to physically shaking him. This same partner was then called by the youth, a few days later, to attend to his mother (with whom he lived) in the middle of the night, on account of what sounded over the telephone to be an acute abdominal emergency. Having misgivings about what situation she might find, and being somewhat fearful of the reception that might await her, she gritted her teeth and made the visit. The mother was indeed in acute pain and there were physical signs of acute appendicitis. This in fact was the diagnosis, as revealed at operation, and after surgery she recovered uneventfully.

Henry did not attend the surgery for the next eighteen months. When he did it was on account of a genuine but minor skin condition and he was able to express gratitude to the doctor for the latter's treatment of his mother. What also emerged was that Henry's father, who was deceased, had always discouraged any show of weakness or sickness in his son, threatening him with (although rarely delivering) corporal punishment. He had therefore never been allowed time off school even for genuine illness. He had viewed doctors as just like his father and, collectively, the doctors themselves had felt increasingly unsympathetic, as the father had been. It was the fortuitous appendicitis in the mother that indirectly resolved the conflictual situation by revealing to Henry a more sympathetic side to the doctor.

As discussed in Chapter 3, a psychodynamic perspective on clinical transactions can aid an understanding of the effect of individuals' past relationships, most notably with parents, on their current relationships, including the doctor–patient interaction. The more the past relationships were based on power and control, rather than on love and acceptance, the more later relationships will bear this same trademark. The more inconsistent and unpredictable are the experiences in childhood, the less will be the capacity to form secure attachments and mature and appropriate dependence and trust in later life. Specific untoward influences, for example, sexual or physical abuse, may leave a particular imprint. In later life the legacy may be addiction, an eating disorder, a sexual perversion, sexual victimisation (as opposed to being a sexual victim) or other personality abnormality, sometimes amounting to personality disorder (Brier and Zaidi, 1989; Herman *et al.*, 1989; Raczek, 1992).

Because of the sense of strain, depression and anxiety caused by an illness and its other secondary effects (for example, loss of earning power), patients may not be able to function at their usual or optimal level of psychological and social maturity. In the presence of a doctor, therefore, the patient may feel as vulnerable as a child. Depending upon the actual childhood experience, and the degree to which psychological maturity (i.e. a capacity to establish mature dependent relationships or secure adult attachments) has developed, childhood experiences or memories may be recalled or emotionally relived. Under such circumstances, the patient may be aware (i.e. conscious) of feeling like a child again and, perhaps, also be able to cope with such feelings evoked by the situation and, in spite of them, play the role of patient adequately, via presenting a complaint and receiving advice, reassurance or treatment, as appropriate.

For patients whose early experience of parents and authority figures was particularly adverse, regardless of the precise details of the adversity, the 'as if' quality of feeling like a child again in relation to the doctor, may be partially or totally lost. Patients may thus feel, at least transitorily, that they are actually in a relationship with former authority figures, now personified by (the person of) the doctor. Thus they may, in effect, present themselves as the complaint, expecting the doctor to deal with 'it'. If asked specifically, such patients, unless frankly psychotic and deluded, would know that the doctor was not in fact the parent.

Much of individuals' perception of others depends upon what they already know or have previously experienced and learned and the consequent working models of the self and expectations of other people that have become established. In that sense, perception is an active, rather than a passive, process. What is known about somebody before they have been actually encountered influences, at least initially, how they are perceived. Considered psychodynamically, the perception and evaluation of another person involves *projective* and *introjective* processes. Projection refers to the process by which specific impulses, wishes, aspects of the self are imagined to be located in some object (including another person) external to oneself. Introjection, by contrast refers to the transposition of objects and their inherent qualities from the 'outside' to the 'inside' of oneself.

On meeting another person, therefore, the subject projects on to that person what is already known. (Such a phenomenon accounts for 'love at first sight', which, at least initially, has little or nothing to do with what the loved person is actually like as a person). The other person in the relationship reacts (consciously and unconsciously) and the result is introjected into the subject's mind and, as it were, compared with the original projection for an evaluation of accurate fit or mismatch. If no mismatch is recognised, then the next stage in the encounter between the two is for the subject to continue to perceive the other in the same way and to maintain the original projections. Most of this processing is carried on unconsciously. If the introjected 'image' (referring to the whole range of personal characteristics, not simply visual) is assessed as different from that originally projected, then, in the subsequent stage of the interaction, the reprojected image differs from the original. In this way, a given relationship may allow each participant to gain a more accurate and complete picture of the actual other person.

In the context of the doctor–patient interaction, involving a patient with a past history of habitual adverse experiences with authority figures, especially when doctors and patients are new to one another, what will be projected on to the doctor may be a condensed image, or caricature, of all the previous parental and authority figures. Under these circumstances, the result will be the perception of a doctor who is imbued with negative attributes – authoritarian, harsh, frightening, seductive, manipulative, insincere – depending upon the perceived quality and experience of the past adverse experiences. Insofar as this projective–introjective process is unconscious, patients will react more to their own projected images than to the real doctor. This obtains unless or until introjected (and sequentially reprojected and reintrojected) images of the doctor are modified in the light of evidence provided by the relationship, as this unfolds, revealing that the actual doctor does not share the characteristics (or, at least, not all of them) of the originally projected image. The more adverse individuals' experiences in their formative years, the more reality distorting are the defence mechanisms employed (see Chapter 3). The result is greater difficulty with perceiving and evaluating the other person in a realistic light.

Transference and countertransference

The above projective and introjective processes involved in the relationship between doctor and patient are carried on at great speed and influenced by verbal and non-verbal behaviour. Much information is thus speedily conveyed and processed. In this sense, the personal level of the interaction is carried out at a much faster pace than that of the public level. Since it is largely unconscious, it is much less available for actual negotiation or discussion than is the public level interaction.

Within psychodynamically informed psychotherapy, the term 'transference' is used to refer to the unconscious displacement on to the therapist of feelings and ideas that derive from previous relationships (Freud, 1912). Much of psychotherapeutic work with patients concerns the clarifying of such unconsciously projected images and facilitating their conscious assimilation. The patients thereby become more insightful into their own mental mechanisms and the way in which their perception of, and relationship to, other people was biassed by their projections.

In relating to their own projected images, more than to the actual other person (i.e. not to introjected and reintrojected images that differ from those they projected), the quality and stability of their relationships is impaired. This is because the relationship is not between two actual people, since differences between projected and introjected images have been denied, ignored or minimised (through the effect of psychological defence mechanisms). With increasing insight, and consonant conscious changes, often in practice meaning the need to endure uncomfortable uncertainty (caused by an acknowledgment and acceptance of the difference between projected and introjected images), patients enter into a more authentic relationship with their therapist. The successful psychotherapeutic relationship is increasingly between two accurately perceived and perceiving people and, as a consequence, its quality and stability is enhanced. The relationship between the therapist and patient matures thus and the patient uses the insights obtained, within the therapeutic relationship, to generalise to other relationships in life.

The interactive nature of all human relationships dictates that each participant is involved in the projective and introjective processes just described in terms of transference. Doctors, too, will therefore project images on to their patients, their *countertransference* (Freud, 1910). Doctors will project images on to a new patient. In such a situation the origin of such projections includes what the doctor may have learnt consciously about the patient, for example, via old case-notes, as well as how he or she perceives the patient when they meet. Like their patients, doctors will be involved in consciously and unconsciously reacting to what they perceive in the other person. The interaction proceeds with multiple projections and introjections, carried out at the personal level, while at the same time the clinical work of the public domain is also being undertaken.

Most often the personal interaction between doctor and patient continues unconsciously and in a manner that supports the clinical goal-oriented activity of the clinical transaction – the public domain. At other times, however, the personal level interaction may fail to support the public domain work of doctor and patient and/or erupt into it. This may result because: (1) doctor and patient fail, in their unconscious negotiation, to agree a personal interactive style and ensuing struggles have a disruptive effect; (2) what is negotiated unconsciously, although stable, results in one participant enacting a psychodynamic pole that is intrinsically opposed to healthy care-seeking or care-giving behaviour (sometimes difficult to distinguish from the first point above); (3) unconscious negotiation is successful, with each participant taking up and enacting a psychodynamic pole that is not obviously or immediately disruptive but that actually is, or insidiously becomes, so. The following clinical examples are used to examine the psychodynamic mechanism of each of these difficulties within the personal interaction between doctor and patient.

Miss Green, a young woman in her teens, presented for advice regarding contraception. She had hoped to discuss this with her usual female doctor, who turned out to be on leave at the time. Only a locum, male doctor, who did not know her, was available to see her. The patient, having steeled herself to consult her usual doctor, appeared to be overwhelmed with embarrassment and fright on seeing the locum. She stared at the floor and remained silent in spite of repeated invitations to talk. The locum doctor, who prided himself on being able to relate to young patients, especially 'difficult' adolescents, felt increasingly thwarted by the lack of a response to his entreaties and ended up exasperated and raising his voice. In response the young woman fled the room.

In the above instance, the doctor responded to a timid and embarrassed patient in such a way as to induce in her more of the same inappropriate care-seeking behaviour. As a consequence, the goal of the clinical transaction was not even established. (It became clear what this had been only after the patient's usual doctor returned and was asked to see Miss Green on a home visit. She had retreated to bed following the consultation referred to above.)

The doctor's response to the patient was, in a sense, *complementary*: she was afraid and he became frightening, at least via his intonation and the loudness of his entreaties. However, this outcome was but one of many possible outcomes. At least in theory, the doctor could have been more

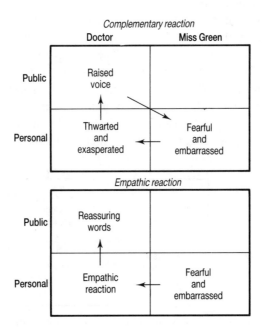

Figure 4.1. Transaction windows indicating that the doctor might have avoided a complementary reaction to Miss Green if the response had been empathic.

sympathetic to his silent patient or, indeed, empathic (Figure 4.1). Had he been empathic then his personal reaction to this patient would have been such as to make him feel upset and awkward, reflecting the introjected image (consciously identified with) of somebody embarrassed and frightened. Recognising and acknowledging such feelings in himself, he might have been able to consider further his emotional response and how he might react. In the event, it may be conjectured, the doctor introjected the patient's obviously awkward predicament but, for personal reasons of his own, could not consciously identify with it. Unconsciously, he became identified with the opposite (the frightener) pole of the psychodynamic (frightener–frightened) theme and enacted it.

The example of Henry, with whose situation the chapter began, is also one in which the doctor(s) enacts a complementary psychodynamic pole that, in this instance, becomes stabilised over time and obviously disrupts the public level interaction, resulting in a complicated clinical transaction. Had the doctors been aware of the phenomenon of countertransference they might have examined their own negative reaction in relation to Henry and attempted to explore, in a more directed way, the psychosocial situation (especially his relationship with his parents), including the doctor–patient interaction at the personal level (transference–countertransference relationship). Had they done so they might have discovered parallels between their own relationship with Henry and that between himself and his father (Figure 4.2). The doctors were clearly aware that all was not well with the clinical transaction. However, being unaware of the phenomenon of the transference–countertransference relationship, they were inevitably caught up in maintaining the status quo and contributing ultimately to an ugly and potentially dangerous escalation. It was only by chance that the doctor–patient relationship was retrieved

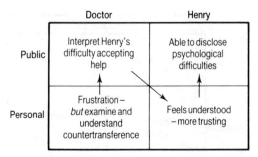

Figure 4.2. Transaction window of the clinical transaction of the doctor and Henry, indicating how an examination of the countertransference permitted interpretation of Henry's difficulties, unlocking the stalemate.

and that subsequent clinical transactions with Henry were more straight-forward.

A newly qualified practitioner, with a professed interest in an holistic approach to patients, became involved in a psychological exploration of a young woman patient, Ms Makin, who presented for a minor gynaecological symptom but, incidentally, divulged a problem to do with sexual dysfunction. The patient, who became increasingly anxious and depressed, needed (in the view of her doctor) an increased frequency of consultations. She professed deep gratitude for the care offered her and, in spite of the increasing psychological disturbance, the sessions continued. Although he experienced the work as arduous, the doctor felt a deep sense of personal satisfaction. After six months had elapsed, however, the patient's dependence upon her doctor had increased to the point that she now telephoned him at home, most evenings and every weekend. Although initially happy enough to accept such out of hours calls, the doctor eventually became abruptly hostile, culminating in his taking the patient in his own car to the local psychiatric unit and demanding in-patient admission for her (Figure 4.3).

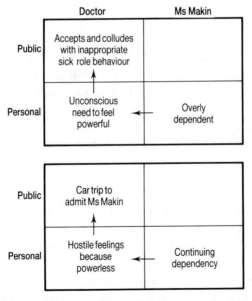

Figure 4.3. Transaction windows of the clinical transaction between the doctor and Ms Makin, indicating how the doctor's personal reaction to her led to her admission to hospital.

Initially, the doctor responded to his patient without a conscious sense of strain or considering the clinical situation to be in any way inappropriate. What was revealed, via the full psychiatric history and family interview carried out subsequently by the admitting psychiatric team, was the fact that the patient's father had grossly indulged his daughter. Mother, on the other hand, was seen to be a driving and capable woman who was emotionally rather cold. She was sexually unfulfilled by her husand yet prepared to stay in the marriage and seek fulfillment through her career. Father felt inadequate and impotent and, partly as a way of gaining daughter as an ally against his wife, indulged her (buying her a fast car and frequent foreign holidays). In this way the patient remained living at home, although becoming increasingly ambivalent about this. Staying at home was also reinforced by the absence of a current satisfactory sexual relationship in her life.

The patient's passive and dependent behaviour elicited an infantilising and active response from her doctor. This was a response that initially made the doctor feel powerful, because of the patient's professed gratitude, but it fulfilled an unmet need for him, as had the daughter's inappropriate dependence for her father. In this example, once more the doctor became involved, unconsciously, in complementing his patient's attitudes and behaviour. Again, the process of the clinical transaction was impaired and the main clinical goals seemingly ignored.

It is very easy for such a complementary response to become enacted because, unconsciously, it suits both parties. It is as if silently each has negotiated a mutually acceptable personal goal, although not necessarily compatible with that of the public domain responsibilities and activities. The more the interaction is positive or neutral in emotional tone, the more it is potentially problematic, since the doctors involved are then less likely to question the appropriateness of their own actions.

Empathy

What emerges from a consideration of the above clinical examples is that success at being in, or sustaining, an empathic relationship (i.e. a concordant as opposed to complementary countertransference) with every patient is by no means guaranteed. There are many reasons for this and within a given clinical transaction the precise reasons will vary according to the individuals concerned and the precise emotional contact enacted at the time. As a process, empathy – the power of projecting one's personality into the object of contemplation (*Concise Oxford dictionary*) –

is carried out unconsciously. It cannot be achieved simply by an act of will. However, an awareness of the phenomenon of empathy, knowing that it is an important ingredient of any therapeutic relationship, and being aware that an empathic capacity can be lost, may sensitise the doctor to failures in the area of empathic interaction.

Empathy, in many ways an everyday phenomenon, represents an important aspect of the doctor–patient interaction, since it reflects a travelling of a certain emotional distance together. It is neither sufficient nor necessary in clinical practice but its presence, almost certainly, has a beneficial effect on the process, and hence outcome, of the clinical transaction. As a phenomenon, empathy demands a certain minimum level of sophistication of psychological functioning, from both doctor and patient.

Since responsibility for monitoring the personal level of the doctor–patient interaction rests with the doctor, the focus here is on doctors' empathic responses, although this implicitly involves patients playing their own part in the process. Empathy has to be understood in the context of a relationship, here the doctor–patient interaction and its presence may serve to influence the direction, pace and content of subsequent stages in the process of the clinical transaction. But, first, it is worth while developing further the notion that empathy is a psychologically sophisticated process.

'The power of projecting one's personality . . .' is part of the definition of empathy. The process of projection is deployed by an unconscious part of the mind, as in the case of a doctor visiting a newly bereaved patient, who finds himself almost immediately close to tears in response to the patient's display of raw emotion. He unconsciously and effortlessly makes an identification with the patient without having to think about how to respond emotionally.

However, empathy also implies the capacity to remain aware of one's own identity as another person. Thus, although doctors unconsciously project into their patients, they need also to take back into themselves, in order to re-establish themselves back in their own psychological shoes. This latter process, like projection, is deployed unconsciously. Empathy thus can be seen as employing both projective and introjective psychological mechanisms. Both processes are a feature of normal relating between people and also part of the formative process of adult personality, undergone during childhood and adolescence (see Chapter 3).

The importance of being in empathic contact with a patient is that in so doing it is likely that the personal level of the interaction will better support the public level and thereby maximise the likelihood that overt clinical goals are secured. One of the tasks for doctors, in monitoring the personal level of interaction, is therefore to recognise their counter-transference reactions to their patients and, especially when this is complementary rather than empathic or concordant, to find a way of understanding this reaction as a 'communication' from the patient.

Countertransference as communication

Returning to the example of the doctors who became negatively engaged with Henry, it might have been possible, at an early stage in the clinical transaction, for one of them to consider why the feelings of frustration were so strong. They could have registered their shared view of him and this might have shed some light on the matter via discussion and they might have attempted to understand what unconscious communication the patient might have been making.

What tends to happen when two people meet is that they search, more or less consciously, for what is a familiar topic of mutual interest or concern. At a deeper level, and carried on unconsciously, they will each be attempting to negotiate a style of relating to one another that can secure, for each of them, the satisfaction of their unconscious needs at the time. Sometimes, such negotiations will be completed quickly and at other times the process may be protracted before finally it precipitates out into a more or less stable relational style. Clearly not all styles are conducive to the successful pursuit of the public level of the doctor–patient interaction. For individuals who experienced adverse parenting and poor quality relationships with authority figures, their familiar response and expectations will often be negatively toned. This familiar response, therefore, is what they may be unconsciously seeking and conveying, via a projected negative image, within the doctor–patient relationship (because this negativity is all they know), in spite of the overt, public level reasons for consulting the doctor.

Doctors must therefore be alert to the emotional replaying of past relationships within the context of their relationship with patients. Important information about the quality and nature of such past relation-ships, largely unconsciously, is being communicated to them. The extent to which they are able to refrain from responses, which fit in with patients' unconscious needs to be maltreated, the more doctors will 'contain' patients' distress and anxiety and this will be experienced by patients, ultimately, as a relief (see also Chapter 7). However, the doctor's capacity for containment may be tested and it may be that the patient repeatedly attempts, often completely unconsciously, to manipulate the doctor into enacting one pole (complementary to the one enacted by the patient) of the dominant unconscious psychodynamic theme of the patient's psychopathology. Paradoxically, patients may be attempting, unconsciously, to push the doctor into a complementary contertransference relationship with them, rather than an empathic or concordant one, in which they may feel respected and understood as individuals in their own right.

An examination of the above issues, in discussion with a patient, may not only serve to increase the latter's personal insight but may also enhance his or her capacity to perform the sick role more appropriately. However, it is quite inappropriate to discuss such matters in all situations or with all patients. These issues of technique, when, how and which aspects to discuss are described more fully in Chapters 6 and 7.

Conclusions

The habitual unconscious deployment of certain defensive strategies, present in varying degrees in both doctor and patient, may profoundly affect and undermine the public interaction, so producing a complicated clinical transaction. This derives from the effect the defence mechanisms exert on the individual's sense of self and others and the resultant working model of self and expectations of others that is set up. At worst the two participants become polarised in attitude and each takes up a complementary, which may often also mean an opposing, position. Such a situation represents a failure of empathy, at least until the emotional reality of the transference–countertransference relationship can be understood. The concept of the transference–countertransference relationship, when applied to the personal interaction of doctor and patient, can illuminate disturbing psychodynamic themes that have been unconsciously and defensively set up, within the doctor–patient interaction, largely in response to the rekindling of interactive styles reminiscent of earlier relationships with authority figures. An understanding of such phenomena and processes can facilitate the doctor in breaking the interactive cycle that maintains polarised and polarising stalemate. In this way the complicated clinical transaction can be returned to the straightforward.

An awareness of the psychodynamic basis of the doctor–patient interaction can alert the doctor to the differing emotional tones and echoes of the dominant psychodynamic theme(s) of the patient's working models of self and other people. These can be viewed as communications and they provide the doctor with an insight into the patient's past, and often also his or her current, important relationships. Thus, being caught up in a complementary countertransference reaction can yield useful information that can be used by the doctor to break the stalemate and to act as a pointer to questions that might form part of a psychosocial enquiry into the patient's network of current relationships (see Chapters 5 and 6).

5

Contextual influences

Introduction

Miss Lake attends complaining of a third episode of sore throat within the period of a year. Before making the appointment she had had an argument with her mother, a chronic invalid, who told her there was nothing wrong with her. Under other circumstances Miss Lake might have struggled on, but fed up with her mother's demands and stung by her lack of sympathy, she presents herself to the doctor in pursuit of the barely conscious goals of getting the sympathy she feels she deserves and at the same time arming herself for revenge on her mother with the proof that she is genuinely ill.

Clinical transactions between patient and doctor do not take place in a vacuum. Each participant is influenced in sometimes subtle and, at other times, penetrating ways by factors that have their origins in contexts external to the transaction itself and may serve to make it complicated. Of these contexts, multiple and overlapping, within which doctor and patient operate, some will be shared and others not. Community, race, gender, social class, position in family, for example, all form contexts that may bring influences to bear on patient and doctor in terms of the dynamics of their interaction. At the public level these might include the shared values and expectations conferred by the social roles of doctor and patient. But those expectations and values will themselves be modified in quality and degree by the personal contexts of each participant, by any idiosyncratic, eccentric or unconventional aspects of doctor and patient as individuals.

Social role theory and psychodynamic theory, even together, cannot describe fully the complex psychological processes that go on within and between individuals as they interact. The clinical transaction occurs within a network of multidimensional contexts. Consequently a theory is required that can inform a method of examining, organising and linking information deriving from, and complementing, the social and psycho-dynamic perspectives. After all, the context is not a random aggregation of people and events but is defined by a relatively obvious and under-standable connectedness, such as a race, culture or family. A context in this sense can be thought of as a system and a theory of systems can usefully be applied.

Systems theory

A system is 'a whole composed of parts in orderly arrangement according to some scheme or plan. A set of assemblage of things connected, associated or interdependent, so as to form a complex unity' (*Shorter Oxford English dictionary*). In biology, sociology and other related sciences the notion of a system has taken on a more restricted and technical meaning (von Bertalanffy, 1973) and systems have been divided into two main types, closed or open. A closed system is, at least theoretically, independent of its environment. Its initial condition is predetermined and, like a battery cell, it can be said to go flat once it reaches its steady state. In contrast an open system is in constant contact with its environment through processes of dynamic exchange, by which it actively attempts to maintain a steady state (homeostasis). The biological cell provides a good example of an open system and all systems that comprise persons are also potentially open systems (see below).

Boundaries, feedback and communication

The dynamic exchange of a system with its environment occurs across a boundary. In the case of a cell, this boundary is its membrane. The internal equilibrium of the cell depends upon its boundary remaining intact. The intact cell membrane exerts some control over the amount and rate of exchanges with its environment. Like other boundaries, the cell membrane is not equally permeable to everything. It lets some things in but not others. Similarly, only some things are allowed out. Some things it lets in at some times but not at others. In other words it is selectively permeable. This function of the cell membrane is, of course, of vital importance in the homeostasis of the cell.

Crucial to the homeostasis (and hence goal, see later) of any open system is its capacity to monitor change both within the system itself and outside in the environment with which it interacts. This implies the existence of a control system and in this respect the notion of feedback is of central importance. Only through a process of error-correcting feedback can the desirable equilibrium of the open system be maintained. In the broadest sense, the exchange and processing of information constitutes the system's communication with its environment. In the case of person-systems the exchange is emotional, intellectual and behavioural.

The output of one system can act only as an input to another if the boundary of the latter system is permeable to it. Thus, the potential inteactions between two systems are seen to be of three kinds (Agazarian and Peters, 1981). First, if neither system is permeable to the output of the other, they may react, but no change in either system will ensue (Figure 5.1, top). Second, if only one is permeable to the output of the other, then the first may change dependent on the output of the second, but not vice versa (Figure 5.1, middle). Third, when both systems are permeable to the output of the other, both may change as a result of their interaction (Figure 5.1, bottom). Such interdependent interaction permits information to be exchanged and genuine two-way communication to occur.

Hierarchies, overlapping systems and isomorphism

The environment of a system may itself constitute a system. In this sense the cell, for example a liver cell, is a subsystem of a larger system, the organ of the liver. The organ is itself part of a larger system still, the body as a whole. Such an arrangement is described as hierarchical.

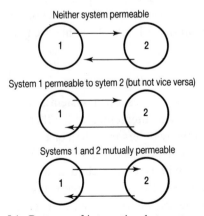

Figure 5.1. Patterns of interaction between systems.

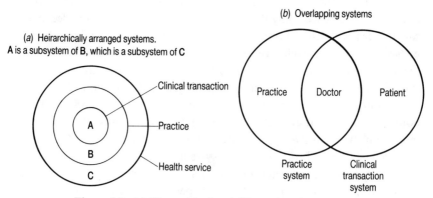

Figure 5.2. (*a*) Hierarchical and (*b*) overlapping systems.

Importantly, the processes occurring at one level may act as inputs to other levels (higher and lower), thus affecting operations at those levels. The effect may be demonstrable throughout the entire hierarchy of systems. If a given system has as one of its members a subsystem that is simultaneously a member of another system, then the systems are said to overlap. Thus the doctor is a subsystem of both the system of the clinical transaction and of the primary care setting itself (Figure 5.2(*a*)). In this respect, the primary care setting and clinical transaction are overlapping systems (Figure 5.2(*b*)).

A study of systems in general reveals that they all share common features of structure and operation. In this respect systems are said to demonstrate the principle of isomorphism (Durkin, 1983). Importantly, this implies that a mechanism operating at one level of a given hierarchy of systems, can be seen, albeit at a different level of abstraction, to operate in the same way in all other levels of the hierarchy (see later).

Person-systems

People can be conceived of as open systems, both as individuals, i.e. person-systems, and when interacting with others in a purposeful way. For example, within the two-person system of a child and his or her carer, attachment comprises a complex set of behaviours with the goal of securing sufficient proximity of the child and carer. This has obvious functional value in terms of survival. As with those processes involved in the homeostasis of the cell's internal environment, a control mechanism is necessary. Attachment behaviour may therefore be triggered, in child or carer, by separation or danger and switched off when secure proximity is achieved (Bowlby, 1958). This in-built mechanism operates automatically and is largely unconscious. As described in Chapter 3, attachment can assume different patterns and take on different emotional tones, which, with repetition over time, become incorporated into the developing personality. This process, together with other behavioural and psychological mechanisms (for example, defence mechanisms), which are similarly incorporated, ultimately results in the formation (in effect) of the boundary of the person-system. Like the membrane of the biological cell, this boundary is selectively permeable. People are more or less thick-skinned – more or less easy to 'get through to'. Doctor and patient, when engaged in negotiating goals relating to health, i.e. enacting the roles of doctor and patient, create another two-person system – the clinical transaction.

Boundaries as barriers to perception and understanding

Doctor and patient perceive each other in a dynamic and selective way, in a sense negotiating a view of each other. This process significantly affects the quality of their interaction and can influence the outcome of the clinical transaction and whether it is straightforward or complicated. The selective permeability of the boundaries between them is determined, in part, by both public and personal domain factors. For example, most doctors will have patients for whom, it seems, they can do no wrong. The patient appears to be sometimes embarrassingly blind to the doctor's imperfections. On the other hand, it can come as a disconcerting surprise to find that a patient who seemed in the consultation to be sensibly co-operative, has not, in fact, complied with the treatment prescribed. In such cases it is as if the expectations of the respective ideal roles of doctor and patient have acted as a filter to remove any evidence that doctor or patient might be unreliable in some way.

Take the case of Mr Crown, the large man demanding an antibiotic (p. 23). The doctor in this instance might have certain expectations of him because of the patient's itinerant life-style, perhaps that he will be demanding and seek to use the service inappropriately. A registered patient, on the other hand, particularly a favourite might have been fitted into a busy clinic list as an extra, without demur. For his part Mr Crown's expectation might be that he is only likely to get what he feels he needs by exerting pressure of a certain kind. To the extent that both are predisposed to view the other according to these, largely stereotypic expectations, they will be less permeable to contradictory evidence; for example, that Mr Crown is at most times a responsible patient and genuinely distressed in this instance, or that the doctor, although time-pressured, is in fact ready and willing to treat. Stigmatic labelling (see Chapter 1) thus represents a circumstance in which boundaries between patient and doctor become particularly impermeable or at least only highly selectively permeable. Personal factors affect communication across interpersonal boundaries and, of course, modify the influence of the expectations of, for example, social role. Thus individuals' expectations of authority figures, based on adverse personal past or current relationships, might well influence their perception of their doctors for the worse.

Construing people as person-systems emphasises the dynamic nature of the perception of others. This can be viewed as an exchange of information across boundaries. There are, however, barriers to perception and understanding that are not easily crossed. Foreign language is an example, and learning disability, in some cases, another. However well disposed doctor and patient are to one another, such barriers may pose real problems for both and may serve to complicate the transaction. Of a different nature is the deliberate use of language to conceal or confuse, as doctors may do by employing euphemism or medical jargon when faced with the task of conveying bad news or dealing with problems at or beyond the limits of their competence.

Goals of the doctor–patient system

The clinical transaction comprises a doctor–patient system that is oriented toward a goal. Goals will vary enormously from clinical transaction to clinical transaction and may not always be what they purport to be. Nevertheless, in general terms, the goal of the clinical transaction might be said to be the alleviation of distress and the maximising of health. Often, within the two-person system of the clinical transaction, the goals of doctor and patient are not in conflict but this ought not to be unquestioningly assumed (see Chapter 4). They each may have subsidiary goals that may not be known to the other or even, in the case of unconscious goals, to themselves. Optimally, doctor and patient, more or less explicitly, negotiate goals for the particular clinical transaction. Such goals may be clearly stateable and are appropriate to the public level of the transaction but they may be unconsciously motivated and refer to personal needs that may not be easily or appropriately brought into the public domain. While they remain hidden or unacknowledged such personal goals have the potential to complicate the public level transaction, especially if they are pursued at the expense of public domain goals.

Roles of the doctor–patient system

In pursuit of the goals of the clinical transaction, doctor and patient adopt roles. If the goal is straightforward and mutually agreed the roles taken will be, at the public level, those of doctor and patient. The roles taken on imply certain tasks for both. For the doctor's part, he or she will be suitably trained and well disposed towards the patient. Expectations of the patient, however, are less clear-cut, largely because of the contribution made by the illness itself to the patient's functioning.

In carrying out their roles, doctor and patient need to balance their internal needs and resources against external demands. The roles adopted will be composed of the relevant skills and attitudes, feelings and behaviour needed to accomplish the tasks in hand. The appropriate skills and attitudes must be selected from the total repertoire in order to play, for example, the roles of doctor, employer, manager and parent appropriately. Those attitudes, feelings or activities that are inappropriate must be suppressed or held in abeyance. For instance, the role of loving partners would not be appropriate in the consulting room.

Each task or goal, together with the role adopted to achieve it, comprises a system with more or less clear boundaries. Success in each role, in terms of its effectiveness in achieving goals, depends on the maintenance of the boundaries of the system. This, in turn, depends on the ability to balance the internal needs and resources of the individual, i.e. the person-system, with the requirements of the environment, in this case the demands of patients, staff, or family. Both doctor and patient can thus be conceived of as being simultaneously members of different systems (either related hierarchically or overlapping with one another) that demand the carrying out of differing roles in the pursuit of the tasks or goals implied by each system. If the roles consonant with one system impinge on those of another that demands a different role, then the transaction can become complicated.

Hierarchical and overlapping systems

A system may itself be included as a subsystem of a higher or super-ordinate system, which in turn may be a subsystem of a higher system still. Thus, doctor and patient, separately, are subsystems of the system of the clinical transaction, which itself is a subsystem of the particular primary care practice. The practice is a subsystem of the primary health care system, which itself is a subsystem of the health service.

Ideally, the goals of higher systems are consonant, if not identical, with the goals of lower systems. The goals are translated into action, however, in different ways depending on the level within the hierarchy. The higher up, the more they are managerial and concerned with planning. Systems lower down the hierarchy are more geared to the implementation of plans, most notably direct patient care of one sort or another.

The doctor's hierarchy

Ideally, the doctor is involved in a dynamic relationship with an environment that places no special demands on the capacity to balance his or her internal needs with the demands of the professional role. Within the boundary of the clinical transaction there should be no conflict between the goals of the transaction as negotiated with the patient, for example a particular treatment for a particular condition, and the goals of superordinate systems of health care. If a conflict does exist, it will create boundary problems between the open system of the individual doctor and higher systems of health care, which may well strain the clinical transaction, thus potentially complicating it and impairing its outcome. For example, at higher levels of health care planning, concern with limiting costs will be a priority. If such concerns cross the boundary of the clinical transaction, doctors may have trouble agreeing to an expensive treatment the patient might require. The doctor may resolve this by redefining particular needs so as to exclude those that cost too much or simply choose to ignore economic constraints. Choosing the former may alienate the patient and the conditions for a straightforward transaction will not be met. Should the doctor choose the latter he or she will stand accused of failing to meet his or her obligations to the rest of society. Either situation is likely to create a conflict of interests that will be reflected in the dynamics of the particular doctor–patient interaction and increase the likelihood that the transaction will become complicated (Figure 5.3). It is quite possible that a given doctor might opt for one solution with some patients and another with other patients and this choice will inevitably be influenced, to a greater or lesser extent, by personal factors influencing the dynamics of the transaction. In any event, in a situation such as this it can be seen that relationships between the various system levels, particularly where goals conflict, potentially exert an effect that may

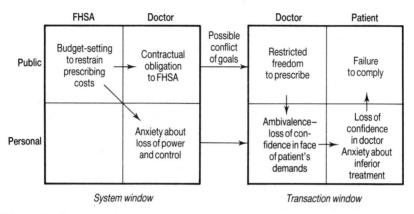

Figure 5.3. System and transaction windows showing interaction between different systems within a hierarchical relationship. FHSA, Family Health Service Authority.

jeopardise the doctor's smooth pursuit of the basic goals of the clinical transaction because of his or her having to manage difficult boundary issues.

The patient's hierarchy

Society's expectations of the patient are less clear-cut than are those of the doctor. Nevertheless, and in spite of the contributions the illness itself might make, the sick role does carry certain expectations (see Chapter 1).

Like their doctors, patients carry on their lives within a hierarchy of systems, multiple and overlapping. As person-systems they belong to family, community and wider society. In many instances the expectations of higher systems will not conflict with the internal needs of patients as person-systems, i.e. the patient is unwell, adopts the sick role and this is accepted by family, workmates, employers and any involved Government agencies. After a defined length of time this role needs the professional endorsement of a doctor. Again, this is often unproblematic. Patient, doctor, family and socioeconomic systems all support a speedy and complete return to health. (Conflict is minimised if there is a clear diagnosis of a disease recognised to cause disability or suffering, particularly if it is visible, such as is the case with a broken and plastered limb. Greater difficulty is encountered when the incapacity is not obvious, as in many instances of mental or emotional suffering or dysfunction, which do not fall easily into any clear-cut diagnostic category and are not easily objectively verifiable.)

Problems can arise if higher systems are, for one reason or another, less tolerant of the sick role. Employers, for instance, may have difficulty coping with the effects of absent workers and exert moral or financial pressure on their workforce not to adopt the sick role even if they feel ill. Within the family, the anxiety and extra workload that looking after a sick family member entails may lead to resentment or the perceived advantage of the sick role may give rise to envy or jealousy. Families vary enormously in their readiness to support a sick member and different patients have different systemic influences, for example having no available carers or being carers themselves. The patient, for his or her part, may be reluctant, at the level of the personal system, to give up the reward (temporary or long-term) of staying ill, for example, the attentiveness of a partner or of a much-needed break from the slog of emotionally and financially unrewarding work. The effect of any of these conflicting goals of hierarchical systems can be to complicate the clinical transaction.

Within a hierarchy of systems the goals of a superordinate system may conflict with those of a subsystem, for example an employer's goal to maximise profits may conflict with a workers' goal to stay home when unwell. Conflict can be more intense if a system belongs, simultaneously, to separate hierarchies. Take the example of the clinical transaction. As a system, it is a subsystem of the hierarchy of systems comprising health care. It is constituted by the person-systems of doctor and patient, who are at the same time members of family and community systems and professional or economic systems. Whereas, ideally, within a hierarchy of systems, goals should be consonant with one another and mutually enhancing, goals of separate hierarchies can easily conflict.

In the case of Miss Lake (p. 67) the locum doctor had no inkling of her covert goals, as she was new to him. Nor had he ever met her mother and thus he was unaware of this contextual aspect of the transaction (Figure 5.4). He happened to be especially concerned with whether to prescribe medication or not, as the use of antibiotics in the particular primary care practice was, at that time, being closely monitored. At a superficial level there was apparent agreement on the goals of the transaction but at a deeper level there was very little overlap (Figure 5.5).

Miss Lake is an integral part of the system of the clinical transaction with her doctor but simultaneously a part of the family system that includes her mother. The overt goal of the clinical transaction is the diagnosis and treatment of her sore throat and, as performing the sick

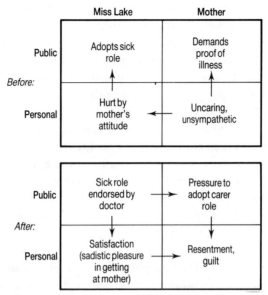

Figure 5.4. System windows showing interaction between Miss Lake and her mother – before and after Miss Lake's visit to the doctor.

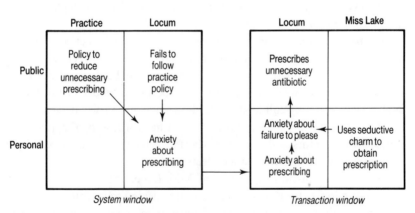

Figure 5.5. Transaction and systems windows showing interactions between locum and Miss Lake and between locum and practice.

role demands, Miss Lake should co-operate and aim for a speedy recovery. The covert goal, i.e. Miss Lake's goal within the family system, is to gain some leverage in the battle against emotional domination by her mother. To this end she may, perhaps unconsciously, wish to feel and appear worse than she is and prolong her illness as much as possible. On the other hand, the locum doctor is, temporarily, an overlapping member of the primary health care team, which, via the auditing of antibiotic prescribing, exerts some constraints on his freedom to prescribe. Thus, if he perceives (in this instance quite accurately) the practice's goal as in some way attempting to limit the prescription of antibiotics, this goal will conflict with some of Miss Lake's covert goals.

The situation might have been further complicated if the usual (non-locum) doctor had been consulted, since he was also Miss Lake's mother's doctor. If such had been the case the doctor would have potentially been a member of two overlapping clinical transaction systems. The doctor might have been aware of the family conflict and have had divided loyalties, fearing that to provide support to Miss Lake too openly might have created a situation of spiralling competition as to who was the sicker and more needy, mother or daughter. The doctor might then have had Mr Lake (Miss Lake's father) telephoning to complain that he could not cope with the burden of his sick family. Although an experienced doctor may be well aware of such complexities, the ability to maintain straight-forward transactions on all fronts may be severely tested. Should the doctor also happen to have unresolved ambivalent feelings towards his or her own elderly, ailing but domineering parent the task might become well-nigh impossible!

The stress of being an on-call doctor in primary care practice is, in part, due to the difficulty of managing boundary issues between work and home. The confusion of boundaries is intensified because, although in some sense still at work, the doctor may be in the midst of the family. Such a situation may call for the rapid alternation of roles depending on the demands of the family (or other social network) and of patients. Of course other factors are also important in this situation, for example, tiredness arising from interrupted sleep.

The above discussion suggests that Miss Lake, at least at times, more or less consciously took on the sick role and elected to maintain it beyond appropriate limits. This may indeed have been the case. In its extreme form, such conscious manipulation of the sick role represents so-called factitious disease or malingering (see Appendix I). However, the sick role may also be adopted unconsciously and be maintained in the absence of conscious motivation. In such situations the sickness may serve a function, not only in terms of the patient's personal needs but also in terms of the requirements of the patient's wider system. For example, a family might, unconsciously, 'select' one of its members to carry the sickness or deviance

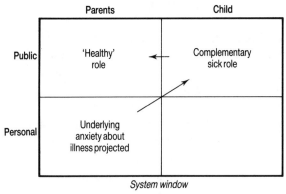

System window

Figure 5.6. System window of a family where complementary roles serve to stabilise the system.

of the family, tending to promote the myth that other family members are free from that sympton. or trait. A sickly child, unable to go out or be left alone, might therefore have a father who is never ill and a mother who, however much she might want to go out into the world, is in fact tied to the home. The personal fears of the parents of illness or the outside, in this way, may be displaced on to the child. By focussing on the sickness of their child, the parents may avoid dealing with their own sickness or that of their marriage (Figure 5.6).

An extreme example of such displacement is found in the phenomenon of Munchausen's syndrome by proxy (see Appendix I). Needless to say, this does not represent the situation in all or even many families with sickly children, or sickly adults for that matter, but, where it does, any attempt to move the sick member out of the sick role threatens the cohesion and homeostasis of the family system and much resistance to change, implied by cure, is encountered. This has obvious implications for the family's relationship with health professionals. (See Chapter 7 for strategies to deal with such complicated clinical transactions.)

Isomorphism

So far the focus has been on problems that affect the interaction of systems, in terms of conflicting goals and roles, and the strain these place on the maintenance of boundaries between systems. Where the integrity of appropriate boundaries is not recognised and respected, transactions may become complicated. What now needs consideration, in addition, is the potentially complicating effect brought about by the phenomenon of isomorphism.

Isomorphism refers to the observation that similar structural and operational features exist at different levels in a hierarchy of systems. Such features, occurring largely outside of conscious awareness, may potentially complicate the clinical transaction. The complication arises out of the effect one level in the hierarchy has on another. This is caused by the transmission of a particular structure or mode of operating at one level that potentially distorts or supplants that at another level. A clinical example may make this point more clearly.

Dr Brown had discovered that a fourteen year old female patient had been sexually abused since the age of six by her stepfather, when he had joined the family. The stepfather was temporarily working away from home and the teenager had not been believed by her mother when she had told her of the abuse. Following this she had taken an overdose of her mother's contraceptive pills. Dr Brown sensitively negotiated with her that social services should become involved. Much to the doctor's surprise the social worker spoken to seemed not to take the matter seriously, indicating that the family was well known to be 'chaotic' and was not able to make use of any help that had been offered in the past. A similar attitude was detected in the policewoman who had been assigned to investigate legal aspects of the case. Dr Brown felt shocked, angered and impotent. She realised, very powerfully, how her patient must have felt not to be believed or taken seriously.

This example illustrates the manner in which a powerful emotional psychodynamic theme in one given system, and at a certain level, resonates and is enacted at another level. In this instance the dynamic between daughter and mother was transposed isomorphically, to the level of the professionals involved in the case. This phenomenon is an important one, not least because knowledge of it can sometimes shed light on what is the key dynamic(s) in the case and sometimes, as in this example, it can have therapeutic value, here, enabling the doctor to be in closer empathic contact with her patient. A dynamic, at one level, that is obscure can be revealed once a dynamic at another level has been identified. In this instance the clearer dynamic (to the doctor) was the one enacted at the level of the professionals. Recognition of this dynamic helped the doctor to identify the dynamic between the patient and her mother. In another example the obscure dynamic might have involved the professionals in the case; then, the dynamic of the patient and family system might have been utilised to shed light on that of the professionals' system.

Complicating factors

Past and current other relationships can exert an influence that serves to distract the doctor or patient from engaging in the tasks appropriate to their public roles, and so complicate the clinical transaction. The doctor in the clinical transaction should, therefore, try to be aware of: first, when feelings and difficulties encountered during interactions in systems outside the particular clinical transaction influence the doctor–patient interactions (in such a situation, the doctor–patient interaction becomes the stage on which is emotionally enacted a drama that rightly should be played elsewhere, for example at the meeting with other professional colleagues, or with meetings with higher management); second, the situation where the opposite occurs, i.e. difficulties arising within the doctor–patient interaction are avoided within the context of the clinical transaction itself and become isomorphically enacted in other overlapping or hierarchically related systems.

As an example of the former, a trainee doctor felt that her trainer, when allocating visits, always gave her a disproportionate number of elderly dependent patients. Although resentful, she felt unable to challenge this, because of her perception of her lower status as a trainee and because she experienced her trainer as rather cold and aloof. As a result, her resentment found expression, not so much in relation to her patients themselves, but through an abruptness and lack of sympathy with their carers. The trainer's attitude towards his trainee, as the carer of his patients, was isomorphically enacted in the trainee's attitude towards the carers of her patients.

Mrs Nugent was a single parent and the mother of two pre-school children. She did not complete her education on account of becoming pregnant and was somewhat resentful of this, the more so because the members of her family of origin were all high achievers, socially and academically. She presented frequently with allergic problems, both on her own account and that of her son who suffered similarly. When seen by either of the two doctors in the primary care practice she was always impeccably behaved. She always took the opportunity, however, to criticise the other doctor, usually on account of any evidence she detected of some, even petty, lack of professionalism. According to her account, for instance, the 'other' doctor had failed to ask her if she was allergic to an antibiotic that she had been prescribed. Criticism became a regular feature of the termination phase of a consultation. In spite of her apparent co-operation, she usually found a plausible reason for not complying with treatment and she would then re-present but, with an uncanny precision, to the second partner. What would transpire was a very similar consultation ending in criticism of the first.

Initially, neither of the doctors related the full story of their own individual interactions with this shared patient and both were unaware of the criticisms levelled at themselves. While they each maintained a friendly relationship with Mrs Nugent, they argued heatedly with each other over her proper management. This argument was fuelled by the barely acknowledged sense of superiority each felt, resulting from Mrs Nugent's criticism of the other. Neither confronted her for criticising the other partner so consistently in spite of her consulting each equally frequently. Interestingly, on most issues concerning medical management the partners could disagree and readily resolve conflicts. Socially, too, the doctors got on very well together. In her interaction with both doctors, Mrs Nugent acted as if the doctor she was with at the time was the 'good' doctor, while the other partner became the 'bad' doctor. The good doctor versus the bad doctor split then became isomorphically enacted in the interaction between the partners. The true state of affairs only surfaced fortuitously when the two of them were talking informally at a Christmas party.

Conclusions

Applying a systemic perspective provides a theoretical framework that can augment both a social role theory and psychodynamic theory view of the clinical transaction. Both public and personal levels of inter-action can be construed as separate, interacting systems. Systems theory emphasises the importance to a system of its boundary. Doctor or patient can be distracted from the straightforward pursuit of the clinical trans-action if boundary issues are mismanaged. This is likely to happen when the goals of interacting systems conflict.

Systems may be related hierarchically, and may also overlap. Ideally, in a system such as an health service, overall goals, and the goals of the subordinate systems within the health service are harmonious. If they are not, the clinical transaction may be adversely influenced and become complicated. On a personal level, where doctor and patient are inevitably members of overlapping systems, individual goals (especially unconscious goals) can easily conflict. Recognising this, doctors can search for the source of difficulty within a clinical transaction as being a manifestation of the conflict between the goals of other overlapping systems, of which they and their patients are members. Constructing transaction and system windows for each overlapping system may help the doctor in this search. Strains at a given level in an hierarchy of systems may pass up and down. The clinical transaction, as a final common pathway and lowest level in the hierarchy, may become complicated as a result.

6

Managing complicated clinical transactions

Introduction

The majority of clinical transactions in primary care settings are routine and straightforward enough to warrant no special attention or modification to their management. The professional relationship seems able to cope with any tendency to wander away from important clinical goals, so that whatever else is also dealt with in the transaction, these are not neglected. But probably at least once in every clinic list the doctor will be left after a consultation with the uncomfortable feeling that something, even if it cannot be exactly defined, was not as it should have been. Sometimes, whole clinic lists can feel like this. Afterwards, the doctor might resentfully think that had it not been for a particular patient all would have been well. Was it, however, the patient's unreasonable behaviour or the receptionist's interruption in the previous consultation or the quarrel before leaving home, that sowed the seed of discontent?

The clinical transaction represents a process that takes place over time, either within a single consultation, or over more prolonged periods and multiple meetings. The doctor must be aware, therefore, of the particular stage of the transaction at any given point, since this bears on the requirements of the interaction (public and personal) at that moment. In the early stages of the transaction, establishing a rapport and a meaningful therapeutic alliance with the patient are important tasks to be addressed. Later, the need to impart information or instructions may take precedence. Later still, disengagement and any associated difficulties with endings may become issues that need attention. To an extent, the shorter the overall length of the transaction the more important are its beginning and ending. During longer transactions there is more room to manoeuvre, to negotiate, to agree achievable goals and to work towards their being secured. Also there is more time for minor departures from the straightforward, particularly within the personal domain, to be corrected, thereby avoiding complication. However, in longer transactions there is more time for goals to be lost sight of and for boundaries to be eroded, the result being a complicated transaction.

Constructing transaction or systems windows, as described in earlier chapters, provides perspectives on the clinical transaction at a given point in time. Being faced with a complicated clinical transaction, and having to decide whether and how to intervene, require a methodical approach. The analysis of complicated clinical transactions is developed therefore using both transaction and systems windows. Postulating the location of departures from the straightforward clinical transaction, taking into account its wider context, suggests possible avenues of returning to the straightforward transaction. Any intervention the doctor undertakes should therefore depend upon an evaluation of evidence for departure from the straightforward clinical transaction. The goal is to return the complicated clinical transaction to the straightforward and, at times, this may entail bringing on to the agenda of the public domain certain aspects of the personal level of interaction. An example might be discussing with the patient the possible reasons for a persistent failure to develop a rapport. It may be necessary to clarify other aspects not ordinarily discussed, such as disagreement between doctor and patient as to the rational basis for a given treatment, arising out of health beliefs that are not shared, or setting limits on what is a legitimate goal for the public level interaction.

As well as departures in the public domain activity, the range of departures from the straightforward clinical transaction includes the following: first, an unduly negative or positive disposition toward the patient on the part of the doctor or insufficient trust and confidence in the doctor or else a too-trusting or over-revealing attitude on the part of the patient; second, inappropriate social behaviour by doctor and patient, i.e. behaviour that is beyond the limits imposed by the social roles of doctor and patient; third, the leakage of feelings (usually negative) on to another system external to the clinical transaction so that those feelings are not experienced as being part of the transaction itself; fourth, the displacement of feelings (again usually negative) from external systems on to the doctor–patient interaction.

In theory, any of the above departures may be directly accessible to introspection by either doctor or patient. In practice, however, such aspects may not be recognised because their presence is ignored or their significance minimised. Furthermore, any of the four departures outlined above may be entirely unconscious to either or both parties. This is particularly likely when feelings are displaced on to or away from the doctor–patient interaction.

Depending upon the precise departure from the straightforward clinical transaction, and the underlying influences producing it, a variety of interventions may be required (see also Chapter 7). It is obviously not possible to outline here all the possible interventions that might be of value nor to give details of where and how they might be deployed. Various strategies are included, however, that indicate the range of responses that might be used when attempting to restore a complicated clinical transaction to the more straightforward one.

In this chapter an overall strategy is outlined and illustrated with the use of flow diagrams. In these diagrams the area in which the departure from the straightforward clinical transaction has surfaced is schematically represented by shading in the relevant pane, and this is indicated in the first box of the flow chart. Each step taken by the doctor in his or her attempt to resolve the complication is then placed in subsequent boxes with arrows indicating the order of steps taken. Without doing full justice to the complexity of the interpersonal interaction involved, such a method is of conceptual value and can be of practical help in unravelling the distressing impasses that complicated clinical transactions often represent. In Chapter 7 more detailed strategic interventions are considered. Both chapters predominantly address the issue of dealing with transactions that have become complicated because of departures that may be conscious or unconscious, within the personal domain.

Public domain evidence

Evidence for departure from the straightforward clinical transaction can become apparent in either domain of the transaction, although this does not indicate the actual source of the complication, as has been discussed earlier. Since each domain affects the other, any public domain evidence of complication may derive from personal domain departures. Therefore, following the discovery of significant departure in the public domain only (for example, failure of treatment compliance), the doctor's *first step* is to examine his or her countertransference reaction and to search for factors in his or her own systems, overlapping or hierarchical (see Chapter 5), influencing the transaction. This first step reduces the likelihood that the patient will be inappropriately labelled as the cause of the departure. Such an undertaking involves the monitoring of any feelings, thoughts, attitudes

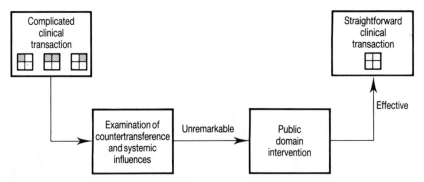

Figure 6.1. Departure in the public domain. Examination of personal and con-textual influences reveals no complications, and a public domain intervention is successful.

or behaviour arising in the context of the transaction, particularly those that seem, on reflection, out of place. If this monitoring reveals nothing untoward, the doctor proceeds with an intervention within the public domain, for example emphasising the importance of complying with treatment, and explaining its rationale, which if successful restores the straightforward clinical transaction. (Complicated clinical transactions, by definition, represent significant and non-transitory departures from the straightforward.) With practice, such an examination of the doctor's personal aspects can be undertaken extremely quickly. The process is illustrated in Figure 6.1.

If, on the other hand, such an intervention, perhaps re-explaining the treatment protocol, should prove to be ineffective, the doctor next examines the patient's personal and systemic influences for any compli-cating aspect, by conducting a *psychosocial enquiry* (see later and also Chapter 9). This requires the doctor to assess and evaluate, among other aspects, the network of social relationships in which the patient participates. Seeking possible impediments leading to the patient's apparent failure to perform the sick role appropriately (here, to follow the treatment protocol correctly) therefore becomes part of the public domain work.

If the psychosocial enquiry uncovers nothing likely to account for the complicating of the clinical transaction, doctors should re-examine their countertransference reactions and any possible systemic influences of their own (Figure 6.2). This may involve looking for major similarities or differences between the patient's and the doctor's psychosocial situations (social class, special interests, religion, culture) and considering, in par-ticular, whether the doctor, in important respects, coincides with a current

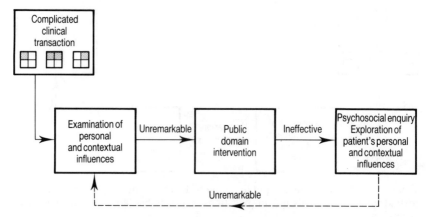

Figure 6.2. Departure in the public domain. A public domain intervention is unsuccessful so the doctor proceeds with a psychosocial enquiry. If this is unremarkable, the doctor re-examines personal and contextual influences.

or past major figure in the patient's life, such as a partner or parent. This should be undertaken *before* returning to a public domain intervention (for example, retaking a history, re-examining the patient, reviewing the differential diagnosis or treatment). Ideally, only after the doctor has considered carefully and resolved as far as possible (and this may involve discussion of the matter with colleagues) any potential complicating factors deriving from his or her own personal domain or systemic influences, should a public domain intervention be tried again. Careful attention to these issues may help to avoid overinvestigation or unnecessary treatment of the patient.

Should the psychosocial enquiry reveal complicating factors in the patient's personal or systemic influences (personal domain) then intervention in either public or personal, or both, domains may be necessary. Such an intervention is aimed at relieving the factors complicating the transaction by resolving any of the patient's adverse personal functioning or systemic influences, including the treating of any diagnosable psychiatric disorder. Should the attention to the patient's personal and systemic aspects prove effective, the transaction may return to the straightforward (Figure 6.3).

This approach is illustrated by the case of Jason, a normally fit and athletic adolescent, who for the first time became wheezy after exercise. His doctor prescribed an appropriate inhaler, explaining to Jason that he suffered from a form of asthma. After two weeks Jason returned, complaining that his breathing difficulties were no better.

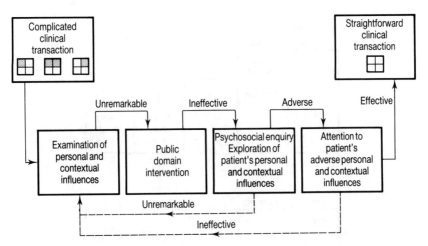

Figure 6.3. Departure in the public domain. A public domain intervention is ineffective. The psychosocial enquiry reveals problems that require attention.

The doctor reiterated the diagnosis, attempted to educate Jason about his condition and checked that he was using the inhaler correctly. (At this point the doctor merely entertained the possibility that the transaction might become complicated.)

Jason went away only to return once more, this time accompanied by his mother, saying that there had still been no improvement. The doctor was now puzzled and entertained the distinct possibility of a complicated transaction, however, she was not unsettled (as far as she was aware having checked her own personal and contextual influences) by the failure of treatment. Nor was the doctor perturbed by the involvement of Jason's mother who seemed appropriately concerned about the situation, since this represented an opportunity to explore systemic influences! Jason's mother asked if the doctor was sure that the diagnosis was asthma and following a brief discussion volunteered that she did not want Jason to take inhalers because she believed they were addictive. She also revealed that she had been asthmatic as a child. The doctor listened to her anxieties and reassured her that addiction was unlikely. She indicated also that Jason's prescriptions would be monitored, as was her routine, so that any such problem could be identified and if necessary dealt with. The mother accepted this explanation and reassurance, and with her support Jason used the inhaler as prescribed (i.e. the potentially adverse systemic influence was corrected) and his asthma responded well (Figure 6.4).

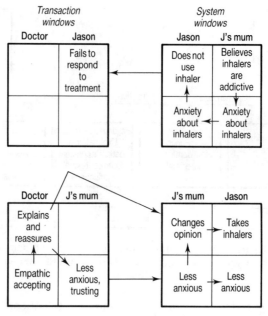

Figure 6.4. Transaction and systems windows of the interactions between doctor, Jason and Jason's mother.

In this example, departure from the straightforward clinical transaction first became evident in the public domain, i.e. Jason's reported failure to respond to treatment. The doctor recognised that the transaction, albeit in an unflamboyant and undramatic manner, had become complicated. (Note: Identifying when a departure from the straightforward clinical transaction has become significant or established is founded on clinical experience and familiarity with the concept of complicated transactions. A complicated clinical transaction, in this sense, does not represent a rigidly definable clinical entity.)

The fact that her reiteration of details concerning diagnosis and advice about treatment went unheeded indicated to her that the departure from the straightforward transaction was indeed significant and non-transitory. On Jason's reappearance, having examined her own personal aspects and taking advantage of mother's attendance, a brief psychosocial enquiry revealed mother's concerns. The doctor hypothesised that it might have been mother's attitude, based on a belief of the addictive nature of inhalers, which interfered with Jason's compliance with treatment, even though this view was not communicated. The doctor's next intervention, which proved effective, entailed education, exploration of anxiety and reassurance and was directed at Jason's mother (i.e. part of his family system).

Personal domain evidence

In certain situations the public level of interaction appears unproblematic but the doctor identifies disturbance in the personal domain. These may be obvious, such as losses of temper, or subtle and only identifiable through close examination of the countertransference reaction. In the latter instance, the only clue may be an uneasy feeling about the quality or content of the transaction, either experienced at the time or in moments of reflection at other times. Alternatively, disturbances in the personal domain may be unconscious and apparently silent and invisible.

There are two main instances of complicated transactions where evidence of departure surfaces in the personal domain interaction. In the first, the doctor's self-examination reveals nothing that might be the source of, or contribute towards, the complication of the transaction. In this instance, the doctor can proceed directly to the psychosocial enquiry, which, if yielding abnormalities, may suggest intervention in the public or personal domain. Should the intervention prove ineffective, the cycle is repeated (i.e. countertransference reaction and the doctor's systemic influences are re-evaluated) and another intervention tried (Figure 6.5).

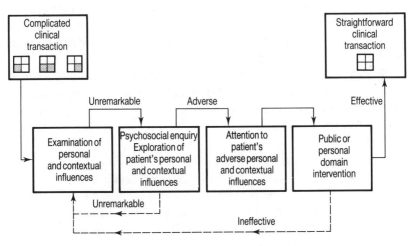

Figure 6.5. Departure in the personal domain. The doctor proceeds with a psychosocial enquiry before attempting an intervention.

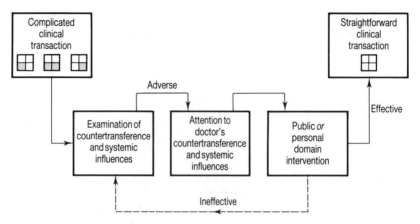

Figure 6.6. Departure in the personal domain. Examination of the doctor's personal and contextual influences reveal problems requiring attention.

Alternatively, the doctor may suspect that his or her feelings and behaviour towards the patient, or the impact of outside influences, are adversely affecting the interaction. In this situation, before doing anything else, doctors should do what they can to remove or mitigate these effects. In the case of strong feelings arising in the countertransference, these may be contained or even brought on to the public domain agenda (see Chapter 7). When recognised, intrusions from external systems, for example conflicts between the doctor and his or her professional colleagues or with the doctor's own family members or wider social network, can then be attended to within the appropriate system rather than through the interaction with the patient. This may be sufficient in itself to restore the transaction to a more straightforward one (Figure 6.6).

Should efforts aimed at putting the doctor's personal and systemic houses in order prove insufficient to restore the straightforward transaction, the doctor proceeds with the psychosocial enquiry of the patient, but only after a further re-examination of his or her own countertransference and systemic influences.

Mr West consulted quite frequently for relief of arthritic pain and sick certification. He accepted treatment and seemed to gain benefit from it but the doctor was always surprised by how tense and angry Mr West seemed to be. The doctor, in response, tended to keep the consultation short and his manner restrained. He also noted his own feeling of depression when he saw Mr West's name on his surgery list. Thinking about this and examining his countertransference, the

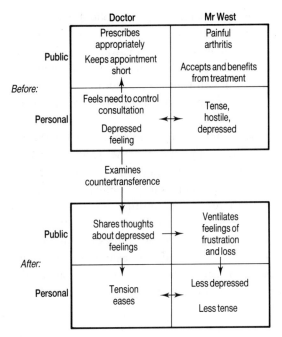

Figure 6.7. Transaction windows of the clinical transaction between the doctor and Mr West, indicating the effect of the doctor examining his countertransference.

doctor tentatively developed two hypotheses: first, that his tight grip on the consultation was almost an echo of Mr West's tension, which seemed barely sufficient to restrain his anger (Mr West gave the impression of being about to explode); second, that the depressed feeling before the consultation might be an empathic reflection of underlying depressive feelings in Mr West. Believing that this was probably a reasonably accurate assessment, the understanding and confidence gained by it made it much easier for the doctor not to simply react to Mr West in a reciprocally aggressive way. Eventually Mr West was able to confess to his frustration and sense of loss arising out of his inability to work. Thereafter the relationship became more cordial, with Mr West attending less frequently and considerably more calmly (Figure 6.7).

Public and personal domain evidence

In many situations, the evidence that a clinical transaction has become complicated appears more or less simultaneously in both public and personal domains. For instance, gross public domain departures such as failure to keep appointments or excessive demands for treatment of minor ailments often go hand in hand with an awareness, if not acknowledgment, that the personal level of the doctor–patient interaction is itself clearly sub-optimal. To deal with transactions complicated in both domains the doctor can deploy a combination of the two approaches developed so far (Figure 6.8).

In essence, the doctor deploys the approach for the *personal domain evidence only* followed by that for the *public domain evidence only*. Because of the interactive relationship between the two domains, it may be that the first approach is sufficient to allow complicating personal aspects to resolve, permitting the public domain departures to heal without specific attention being paid to them. Clearly, in many clinical situations this desirable outcome does not materialise. Should this prove to be the case, then, after re-examining the countertransference and any systemic intrusions, the doctor needs to pursue the psychosocial enquiry and attempt to deal with any problems revealed by it.

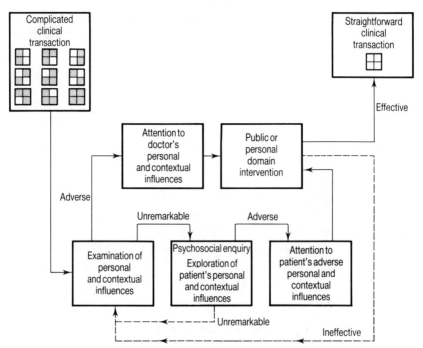

Figure 6.8. Departures in public and personal domains. Procedure for personal domain departure applied first, followed by procedure for public domain departure.

Important clinically, and probably quite common, is the clinical transaction that is actually complicated on both public and personal levels but in which the only manifest evidence of complication lies in the public domain, for example poor compliance with treatment. Examination of countertransference reaction will have revealed no abnormalities but this will have been achieved only by the doctor having rationalised that any bad feelings he or she might experience, for example during the actual interaction, really belong outside the transaction. In this way feelings are displaced away from the interaction with the patient and located, perhaps with seemingly good reason, in other 'external' systems (for example, that of health services management, other medical colleagues or the reception staff). Such feelings, of course, should be identified through a consideration of contextual systemic influences but this may not always be the case. Therefore, the doctor should bear in mind that his or her feelings, to whomever else attributed, may not occur with other patients on that day, thus these feelings do actually derive from this particular doctor–patient interaction.

The doctor, therefore, needs to take care to pay particular attention to the examination of countertransference feelings and the influence of overlapping systems. The task becomes one of accepting that those feelings attributed elsewhere (no matter how accurately) do, none the less, belong *also* within the relationship between the doctor and the patient. This entails that boundary or gate-keeping issues, between the system of the transaction and overlapping systems, are monitored sensitively and well. This in turn depends upon an awareness that mechanisms operating within the transaction, at an unconscious level, may resonate isomorphically and become enacted in other systems of which the doctor is a member (see Chapter 5, Mrs Nugent whose doctors both saw themselves as 'the' expert on her case).

Another relatively common example of this complex state of affairs is represented by the case of Mrs Jones. Her doctor had referred her for a surgical opinion because of recurrent bouts of abdominal pain. He, himself, had attributed her pain to an irritable bowel but persistent and various efforts at treatment had proved unsuccessful. Mrs Jones, in spite of her repeated complaints, had a lively demeanour and the doctor privately acknowledged he felt a definite sexual attraction towards her. The presentation of her symptoms seemed genuine and although her doctor enquired about possible emotional or stress-related causes which might account for exacerbations of her symptoms, these were denied and, indeed, were belied by her appearance.

Inwardly, the doctor expected little to emerge from the specialist referral. After seeing the specialist, however, Mrs Jones returned to complain in an uncharacteristic angry, bitter tone, that the specialist had 'barely looked at her' before telling her there was nothing wrong.

The doctor was aware of feeling some anger with the surgeon on behalf of his patient. The latter went on to say that she now had to attend the hospital for a barium enema. The doctor mollified her and she left seemingly quite cheerful. However, the enema proved to be an awful experience for Mrs Jones and she was again furious with the specialist's abrupt manner and uncaring attitude when he told her that no pathology had been found and discharged her promptly from the clinic. Feeling angry himself at this apparently discourteous and disrespectful behaviour on the part of his specialist colleague, the doctor said he himself would inform the hospital as to how Mrs Jones had experienced her investigative ordeal. Mrs Jones left after a cheerful and friendly exchange at the end of the consultation.

What merits attention, in the case of Mrs Jones and her doctor, is the way in which their 'good' relationship was preserved in spite of the doctor's own failure to relieve her symptoms. Not only did he fail to ameliorate her symptoms but indirectly he subjected her to a series of encounters and investigations which she experienced as painful and deeply humiliating. The anger that was felt by both Mrs Jones and her doctor was directed at the hospital system and seemed to be entirely absent from their own interaction (the system of the clinical transaction). For his part, Mrs Jones' doctor felt little frustration with her failure to respond to his efforts to treat her. Furthermore, after her outburst of anger, which after all was directed at the specialist of his choosing, he immediately sided with her against his colleague. Speculatively, this may have been motivated by guilt (conscious or unconscious), not only for putting his patient through her ordeal but also for wanting to avoid a lengthy explanation of her condition and detailed exploration of its potential psychosocial aggravants. Mrs Jones' reaction might have been fuelled by an unconscious anxiety and anger arising out of a sense of being let down by her doctor's inability to cope with her and her symptoms, in effect experiencing this as a rejection.

It is likely, in this case, that Mrs Jones and her doctor preserved their relationship by splitting (unconsciously compartmentalising) good and bad feelings with the result that the bad feelings were denied within, and displaced outside, their relationship. In this particular case the fact that Mrs Jones presented persistent symptoms yet seemed lively and cheerful with her usual doctor, yet was so angry with the specialist, raises the possibility that she prominently deployed immature defence mechanisms as an aspect of her personality. The doctor unconsciously participated, perhaps for psychological reasons of his own, which prevented him tackling a complex clinical problem, his preference being to preserve a good relationship with an attractive patient. He might have been more questioning of her expectations of the referral to the specialist and her interpretation of events, not so readily relinquishing his own good opinion of the surgeon (see Figure 6.9).

It is not uncommon for doctors in primary care settings to refer patients for a specialist opinion when a clinical transaction has reached what is experienced as an impasse, most commonly where patients have a chronic condition and have failed to achieve what they themselves consider to be an acceptable level of health. The doctor may be confident that the referral will not change matters but does not feel able or willing to undertake the sometimes difficult task of explaining to, or convincing, the patient

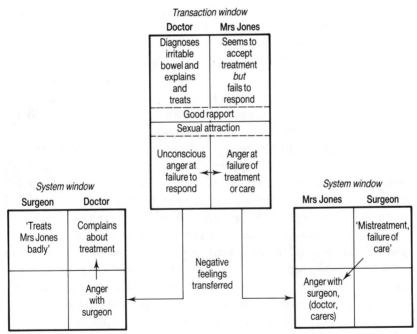

Figure 6.9. Transaction and system windows showing the interactions between the doctor, Mrs Jones and the surgeon.

that this is the case. The effect of the referral is to relieve the doctor of a burden but it may expose the patient to ultimately fruitless, and potentially harmful, further medical involvement.

Psychosocial enquiry

Carrying out a psychosocial enquiry is required in two main situations: when a psychological symptom is presented, and the enquiry is part of public domain activity; or when the clinical transaction has become complicated and a psychosocial enquiry is required as part of an exploration of the patient's personal level contribution to the complication. This applies, as discussed in some detail above, in three sets of circumstances (Table 6.1).

The transition to a psychosocial exploration within the clinical transaction, which is overtly concerned with a physical symptom or disease, often requires some tact and skill on the part of the doctor. However, this transition is itself, in a sense, an intervention and may be approached in a number of possible ways, an example of which described in the next chapter (see Interpretating, p. 109). It must be remembered, however, that each clinical transaction is unique, depending as it does on the relationship between an individual doctor and patient. The relationship may be based on a history of more or less secure and appropriate professional contact, i.e. straightforward clinical transactions. On the other hand, previous contact between the patient and the medical profession may have been quite unsatisfactory on account of any number of complicating factors. Each situation, in a general way, brings with it implications for the clinical transaction and hence for the doctor's approach to it.

What is required, within the psychosocial enquiry, is for the doctor to ask relevant questions, in an appropriate manner, to tease out the patient's personal contribution to the complicated clinical transaction. These fall into three main areas (Table 6.2) and correspondingly questions are aimed at: first, identifying conflicting goals from overlapping systems (for example, Jason was a member of a clinical transaction system with the goal of taking inhalers to control his asthma, and a family system including his mother, whose goal was to stop him using inhalers, out of a fear of addiction); second, identifying attitudes towards past and present significant others, especially involving issues of trust, dependency, power and loss, which contributes to the patient's transference relationship with the doctor (as in the case of Henry and the three doctors, Chapter 4); third, exploring personality organisation (especially to identify

Table 6.1. *Indications for undertaking a detailed psychosocial enquiry*

(1) Evidence arises in the public domain and the doctor's self-examination reveals nothing untoward; yet appropriate public domain intervention proves ineffective
(2) Evidence for a complication arises within the personal domain and any necessary action, based on self-examination, proves ineffective
(3) There is evidence of complication from both public and personal domains

Table 6.2. *Objectives of the psychosocial enquiry*

(1) Identify conflicting goals from overlapping systems
(2) Identify attitudes towards past and present significant others
(3) Explore personality organisation and type

predominance of immature defence mechanisms) and type insofar as it may influence illness behaviour (as in the case of Mrs Jones and her referring doctor).

With certain patients the effect of bringing hitherto hidden personal aspects legitimately into the light of the public domain work may be sufficient to restore the transaction to a straightforward one, as in the case of tense and angry Mr West above (p. 92). Others may be reluctant to admit to psychosocial difficulties, even when these are demonstrably present. Alternatively, they may be reluctant to relinquish a somatic complaint or to give up an embattled or dependent personal relationship with the doctor because it would entail giving up unconscious (primary) or secondary gains. Such situations may demand much of the doctor's skill, patience and time and, once more, in-depth discussion with colleagues may prove to be invaluable.

Contextual influences

The patient will be a member of a number of systems. Usually these will be overlapping rather than hierarchically related. Of particular relevance are the systems of the culture, the family and any work situation. There may be therefore conflicting pressures on the patient, for example to take time off work in order to comply with a particular treatment yet to remain at work in order to safeguard a job or to avoid the difficulties associated with financial loss. Also, conflict may arise from another source, of a different kind but of considerable importance, when health-related beliefs and ideas differ from those of conventional medicine. These may derive from cultural or subcultural influences. It is now well established that lay ideas regarding medicine play an important part not only in the presentation of illness but also during treatment (see Chapter 1). Such a conflict between competing systems of health beliefs, between that of the patient and that of the doctor, can impose considerable strain on the doctor–patient interaction and thereby complicate the clinical transaction.

In order to understand and gauge the importance of potential conflicts of this sort, the doctor must become acquainted with the patient's culture and subculture, particularly where health beliefs are concerned. Even so the doctor may need to explore with the patient, and perhaps with the patient's family, any specific or idiosyncratic attitudes towards illness in general or towards particular symptoms and towards particular treatments or investigations. Clearly, it will also be highly relevant to have some knowledge of the attitudes of the employers and of the patient's working environment that might compromise the patient's ability to perform the sick role appropriately. Only when in possession of this range of information may the doctor fully appreciate the significance of the current illness to the systems within which the patient lives and works.

Relationships with significant others

The quality and style of relationships which the patient brings to the interaction with the doctor may bear the trademark of earlier relationships to authority figures, for example parents, teachers or the police. It is in part through the persisting effect of these relationships that the patient's transference relationship with the doctor is determined. The relationship style with the doctor may also mirror current relationships, perhaps with a boss or sexual partner, since these also often derive from earlier relationships. Obtaining information about other current relationships may therefore indirectly shed light on that of doctor and patient, especially the enactment of complementary roles (see Chapter 4).

The effect of serious physical, sexual or emotional abuse or of neglect, which may be revealed by sensitive history-taking, can have a profound effect on the patient's subsequent ability to relate to the doctor in a straightforward way. This is particularly true if such abuse operated over extended periods of childhood and adolescence and has therefore been instrumental in the development of personality. Thus, eliciting information that relationships were based on power and control rather than on acceptance and love, were marked by a profound ambivalence, or involved unresolved grief following the loss of a parent or carer, may be useful in helping the doctor to construe his or her own current interaction with the patient.

Specific illness beliefs may also be embedded in the relationships with significant others, past and present, and may influence illness behaviour. On occasion, for example, a given patient may have considerable emotional investment in remaining sick. In certain circumstances, therefore, it may be very useful to interview other family members together with the patient to explore such issues. Patients who have been significantly abused or neglected often have later difficulties in trusting and hence becoming appropriately dependent on professionals, including their doctors. They thus have difficulty formulating a complaint and asking for and receiving help (see Chapter 3).

Personality and level of personal functioning

People who habitually deploy immature defence mechanisms, as part of their personality and everyday personal functioning, often have difficulty performing the sick role appropriately. The doctor may already have the skill and experience to recognise the particular style of relating associated with the deployment of such defences or may rely upon a psychiatric opinion to provide this information (see Chapter 3). What is likely to be obvious, however, is the particular type or colouring of the patient's personality: obsessional, paranoid, histrionic, dependent, schizoid, antisocial, etc. (see Appendix II). The effect of illness tends to exacerbate personality characteristics, for example, obsessional patients may become more inflexible or pedantic under the stress of illness. This may have implications for their management (as discussed earlier in Chapter 1). Thus, the obsessional patient may need more notice of investigations or of any changes to the treatment plan and a lengthier discussion giving more detail than does a non-obsessional patient. The schizoid patient may appear to react without emotion to a distressing diagnosis and the doctor may need to go to greater lengths than usual in order to find out what the patient actually thinks and feels.

Doctors' personalities too may have any of the characteristics outlined above with corresponding implications for their behaviour, especially when under stress. For example, an obsessional doctor may become more so when stretched due to chronic fatigue or acute time pressures and make exhaustive, and exhausting, efforts to establish a definitive diagnosis. It may be important therefore for the doctor to build into the working day opportunities for unloading the stress of dealing with the pressure of demanding work (see Chapter 8). Because of the interaction, and to a variable degree unconscious, nature of the relationship with the patient at the personal level, patients with certain personalities will pose particular problems for certain doctors, and vice versa. The interactive effect may produce a complicated clinical transaction.

As part of the psychosocial enquiry, the doctor will need to ascertain the level and quality of current functioning of the patient and be able to contrast this with the patient's usual level of functioning (where this is different) as revealed by appropriate history-taking and, when necessary, seeking after collateral information culled from other sources (the patient's family, other carers or other professional agencies). This approach should bring to light any psychiatric disorder, if present, which may need treatment in its own right, either by the doctor or through referral to a relevant specialist, usually a psychiatrist.

Conclusions

A methodical approach to complicated clinical transactions, as outlined in this chapter, is required for two main reasons. First, to minimise or remove, as far as possible, the doctor's contribution to the complicated clinical transaction via an adverse, unwitting countertransference or systemic influence. Avoiding such a negative effect is achieved by examining thoughts, attitudes, feelings and behaviour, insofar as they form part of the countertransference to the patient or stem from conflicts arising out of incompatible goals of other systems. By so doing, the doctor avoids automatically identifying the problem with the patient. Second, such an analytic approach will usually suggest ways of intervening in the trans-action, for example indicating the area in which an intervention should be attempted, either at the public or personal level of the transaction.

The analytical approach to the complicated clinical transaction, utilising the transaction or systems windows as appropriate, can begin formally, as a paper-and-pencil exercise. It can be undertaken by the solitary doctor or between two or more doctors, including between trainer and trainee(s). Alternatively, it can take place within a small group of doctors specifically looking at complicated transactions (see Chapter 8). This is especially advantageous when complications persist and the doctor does not recognise or acknowledge any personal domain problems. Otherwise, it may be employed in day-to-day work whether or not it is formally recorded using the window methods. Regular use of the approach is crucial to enhancing the doctor's awareness of the process of a clinical transaction and sensitises him or her to early evidence of departure from the straightforward clinical transaction, thereby increasing the likelihood that any complications are corrected before becoming firmly established.

A psychosocial enquiry is required in certain situations. It may help to identify problems arising out of the patient's involvement in family, culture or work, and reveal health beliefs that conflict with those of conventional medicine. It also allows the identification of aspects of personality that may bear on the patient's capacity to perform the sick role and influence the interaction with the doctor, thereby complicating the transaction. This in turn has implications for the doctor's personality and style insofar as he or she may be more or less likely to enact a complementary role, thus becoming inadvertently involved at the expense of the public domain working and goals.

7

Interventions in complicated clinical transactions

Introduction

In Chapter 6 a methodical approach to analysing complicated transactions was developed. In every case, even where departures are only apparent in the public domain, the doctor's initial response is to examine his or her own feelings and behaviour (i.e. countertransference reaction and systemic influences). This initial step is taken in recognition of the fact that any action a doctor takes within a transaction is susceptible to influences other than those of the strictly clinical requirements of the transaction. As discussed in earlier chapters, public and personal levels constantly interact. Public domain departures, therefore, may in fact originate from aspects of the personal domain of the doctor–patient interaction, aspects that may be unconscious or unacknowledged. As a consequence the doctor's actions may at times be motivated, even if unconsciously, by: emotional reactions to the patient arising out of the transference–countertransference relationship; or an attempt to reconcile the conflicting goals of overlapping systems, for example pressure to comply with budgetary constraints; or incompatible (medical and lay) theories about the causes and treatment of illness.

Interventions aimed at rectifying complicated transactions that fail to take the personal dimension into account may result in an exhaustive and fruitless cycle of medical investigation and treatment that fails to address the underlying problem. In addition, there is always the temptation to look first at the patient's contribution to the complication, with a corresponding tendency to hold the patient entirely responsible for any or all departures from the straightforward. As emphasised elsewhere (Chapters 3 and 4), this is particularly likely to happen when immature defence mechanisms are operating in either patient or doctor. The result is often a frustrating deadlock, with the personal level of the doctor–patient interaction gaining inappropriate prominence and providing an emotional environment that feeds on stigmatic labelling – the 'quack' and the 'problem patient'.

When there is evidence of departure from the straightforward clinical transaction in the personal domain, whether or not accompanied by a departure in the public domain, a psychosocial enquiry (into the patient's personal functioning and family and wider social network, i.e. systemic influences) becomes a necessary second step before deciding when and how to intervene in a complicated clinical transaction. In some situations the result of such an enquiry may be that the further management of the transaction becomes more clear-cut, as when a psychiatric disorder is revealed. For example, a depressive illness may be presented somatically, or even via a surrogate patient, and be associated with anxiety or hostility that disturbs the personal level interaction. Further enquiry might reveal characteristic sleep and appetite disturbances, making apparent the diagnosis of a depressive disorder for which anti-depressant drugs may be the first line of treatment. The disturbing personal domain aspect is then dealt with as part of public domain activity. In other situations the approach may be less certain and involve any or all of the interventions discussed below and, no doubt, more besides these.

In all cases of established complicated clinical transactions, the doctor's judgment of when and how to intervene is based on an assessment of the patient that includes the patient's:

(1) family and wider social network influences;
(2) style and quality of past and current relationships with important figures in his or her life;
(3) personality and level of social functioning (including any diagnosable psychiatric illness);
(4) current relationship with the doctor and prevailing mood state.

Note: The overall goal of an intervention in a complicated clinical transaction is to elevate into the public domain any covert, especially personal domain, aspects of the transaction that have resulted in departure from the straightforward. This allows such complicating factors to be more openly discussed within the interaction so that they can potentially be resolved via the continued and collaborative efforts of doctor and patient conforming to their usual, conventional social roles.

Interventions

Interventions by the doctor are, of course, an everyday aspect of any clinical transaction. The most habitually deployed by a doctor are a reflection of his or her usual style of consulting, and can be categorised in a number of ways (for example, see Heron, 1975). They may be motivated and evoked by factors in the doctor–patient interaction of which the doctor may, or may not, be aware. A doctor might, for instance, seek to inform, instruct or educate a patient about his or her illness and its treatment and be more or less confrontational or sympathetic in the process. He or she may be more or less comfortable making an intervention that might, for example, facilitate the release and expression of strong motion of one kind or another. If asked, the doctor could no doubt provide valid reasons, based on the clinical needs of the transaction, for any or all interventions made. But inevitably, the timing, manner and spirit of the intervention will also be underpinned by unconscious aspects of the interaction with the patient, regardless of whether the transaction is straightforward or complicated.

The emphasis in this chapter, however, is on the doctor's options that might be especially useful for intervening in established complicated clinical transactions and that can be deployed in order to carry out the management tasks identified in Chapter 6. Such interventions can, however, be used prophylactically, in order to prevent transactions becoming complicated in the first place, if coupled with the ongoing public and personal domain monitoring of the transaction described in earlier chapters. As noted in Chapter 6, some interventions will tend to be more appropriate and relevant to earlier stages of the transaction and others more to later stages.

Clarifying and elucidating

Clarification and elucidation are everyday features of clinical transactions and form part of any clinical problem-solving approach. The problem as presented by the patient is not always clear-cut. Part of the routine public domain work, therefore, involves patient and doctor negotiating a shared understanding of the problem and its proposed solution. How much sharing, and how much negotiating, depends, among other things, upon the style of the relationship, which in turn is a product of the personal styles of doctor and patient. That this work may prove taxing does not necessarily mean that the transaction has become complicated, since both parties pursue a common, if as yet not precisely defined goal. If the transaction has become complicated, clarification and elucidation may then need to focus on particular aspects of the doctor–patient interaction. Roles, expectations and appropriate behaviours may need to be clarified and, if necessary, strictly defined (see also Setting limits, p. 113). Areas of disagreement over the causes and treatment of illness may need elucidation. As discussed above, doctors will also need to keep in mind the fact that systemic influences (for example, their respective health beliefs or family conflicts) are acting on and influencing both themselves and their patient.

Mr Knight, at the age of fifty-six, had just been made redundant. He had attended the surgery to ask for a 'sick note'. If certified unfit for work he could avoid having to join the unemployment register, which would otherwise entail his looking for and being available for work in order to qualify for benefit. He cited a 'bad back' as reason for his sickness and demanded certification. The doctor, more than a little taken aback, stated that she would not accommodate his request. After all, Mr Knight had been fit enough for work until that very morning – she could not provide a sick note simply because he had been made redundant. Mr Knight, who was an infrequent attender at the surgery and hence unfamiliar to his doctor, angrily expostulated that his back made it impossible for him to work. Feeling annoyed by what she regarded as abnormal illness behaviour, but seeking also to calm the situation, the doctor explained what were her duties and obligations with regard to sick certification. Mr Knight, somewhat soothed by his doctor's restrained and respectful manner, was able to understand her predicament of needing to diagnose before being able to provide sick certification and went on to present the symptoms of his back condition in enough detail to convince the doctor that he did indeed have a genuine problem. The transaction thereafter proceeded straightforwardly. The doctor had, in effect, made an intervention on both levels of the interaction. On the personal level (having monitored her countertransference feelings of annoyance) she acted to defuse an angry stalemate by making her tone calm and reasonable, while on the public level backed this up by clarifying her role, and Mr Knight's expectations of her, in respect of sick certification.

The first of these interventions, arguably the more effective, involved the doctor taking stock of and containing her emotions (note: the concept of containment is discussed below). However, clarifying the respective social roles of herself and her patient (i.e. their respective systemic influences) were undoubtedly also helpful interventions, leading the transaction back to the straightforward. Of course, clarification and elucidation are commonly used by the doctor during history-taking in order to correctly identify and categorise a patient's symptoms as part of public domain activity.

Imparting information

During the course of many clinical transactions some time will be spent educating the patient about the nature, cause and management of an illness. Often it can be helpful for patients to learn not only about the clinical facts but also something about their possible psychological reactions to illness. To hear that an illness is known and understood is reassuring; it is also reassuring for patients to discover that their personal reaction to their illness is understandable to the doctor and something that can be talked about.

A young mother telephoned her doctor having just discovered, at bedtime, that one of her children had worms. She was agitated and distressed, almost in a state of panic, and wanted some form of treatment for her child there and then. The on-call doctor, who had had a long and busy day and had not yet had time for an evening meal, started to tell her that this was hardly an emergency and could perfectly well wait until morning. Becoming aware of his own unfriendly tone, he continued more gently to talk about threadworm infestation, saying that the condition was a common one and her reaction not unusual and that, in fact, there was no immediate threat to her child. After further discussion she was happy enough to delay the consultation until the following day.

In this example it was not simply the apprehension of any physical threat to her child that so distressed the mother but the reaction of disgust and shame on discovering the worms. It was these psychosocial aspects that the doctor hoped to address by his intervention of imparting information. By holding his irritation in check he had allowed this intervention to be effective.

Patients' behaviour and lifestyles may affect the somatic presentation of physical illness and vice versa, in a manner and to an extent of which many patients may be ignorant. Time spent educating the patient about such mutual influences may be appreciated and sometimes sufficient in itself to resolve complications at the personal level of the interaction with the doctor. For example, the patient may not know of the secondary effects of depression, such as low energy, poor sleep and weight loss, which can so impair his or her psychosocial functioning. Or within a family system, it might be that one member's illness or bad behaviour, reinforced by the reactions of other members, has the effect of camouflaging other family problems, which consequently remain unresolved. Pointing out this possibility, of which patient or family may have been unaware, can provide relief, impetus for change and, sometimes, enhanced treatment compliance.

When dealing with, or seeking to prevent, complicated clinical transactions, the approach that may be most helpful often involves making explicit the ways in which illness and the reaction to illness affect the process of the transaction. Anxiety, disgust or shame often impel patients to seek urgent help but may also cause delay in presentation and may make them intolerant of further delay or frustration. Help with separating such feelings from the actual threat of the illness, and at the same time facilitating an open acknowledgment of them, often allows the more realistic implications of the illness to sink in and in this way the likelihood of the transaction remaining straightforward is increased. However, many clinical transactions remain complicated in spite of such efforts on the part of the doctor.

Interpreting

The term 'interpretation', in the context of a complicated clinical transaction, embraces any comment the doctor might make that brings into the public domain aspects of the psychodynamic process of the personal level of the transaction. It may become clear, for example, that what is being enacted between the doctor and his or her patient is a complementary transference–countertransference relationship (see p. 59). On the basis of such an understanding it may then be possible for the doctor, after relevant enquiry, to suggest that he or she is being experienced just as were earlier carers or authority figures in the patient's past life. It might also be possible to acknowledge the doctor's contribution to maintaining this style of interaction, which, in fact, may be inappropriate in the context of the clinical transaction.

The timing and style of delivery of such an interpretation is of great importance. It would be unlikely to be helpful if given when patient and doctor are in the grip of especially intense negative feelings arising out of their interaction. Indeed it might then be quite destructive. Perhaps the most auspicious timing would be during a moment when the patient and doctor can together quietly ponder the impasse that has developed. If delivered in a spirit of enquiry rather than dogmatism, the patient has the option of refuting the interpretation without this too becoming part of any confrontational or argumentative exchange and neither party need lose face.

Mrs Mostyn was increasingly viewed as a real problem for the doctors in the practice. She persistently complained of an unremitting headache and repeatedly demanded to see a doctor. Over the course of many months she had been thoroughly investigated including referral to secondary care specialists but no organic disease had been found. In addition she had become dependent on painkilling drugs. Her tone was petulant and self-pitying and so difficult did the doctors find her that they tended to see her in tacitly agreed rotation. Finally, one of the doctors decided to see her for a longer appointment in the hope that some way could be found to relieve the situation. By this stage all the doctors felt exasperated, hopeless, and barely capable of being civil to her.

During a careful retaking of the history, Mrs Mostyn said that her headaches had started shortly after her son, the last child to leave home, had emigrated to Australia. When asked if she missed him she became tearful and the doctor, who knew nothing of her childhood, asked about other losses in her life. She disclosed that her mother had died when she was only six. This left her, the youngest child by some years, in the care of her father. In fact the caring was taken on by her older sisters who were already married and with children of their own. Apparently they too took it in turns to look after her. Noticing the parallels between past and present, the doctor gently pointed them out, suggesting in some ways she seemed like her childlike self, and the doctors like her sisters, whose patience often wore thin having an extra child to care for. It also became clear that Mrs Mostyn's husband was incapable of coping with his wife's distress and tended to stay out most of the day – much as her father had been out at work and unable to cope with a grieving and demanding child. After a tearful half hour Mrs Mostyn left, agreeing to see a counsellor and to explore her unresolved grief and reassess her relationship with her husband. Over some months with the counsellor Mrs Mostyn improved. She continued her tendency to present with somatic complaints but attended far less frequently and with a greater capacity for insight. The doctor took care to tell the other doctors what had transpired so that they in turn might not continue to be caught up in the complementary transference–countertransference relationship as before.

Mrs Mostyn was able to make use of the interpretation her doctor offered but it may often be the case that patients cannot do so. Interpretations may be wide of the mark, mistimed or delivered inappropriately, but in addition, some patients seem unable to recognise their own emotional states or reactions (see Appendix I: somatisation, alexithymia), or else have too much invested in the status quo to be capable of benefiting from an interpretation. With many patients, however, a simple statement acknowledging or pointing out the recurrent tendency for transactions to end in some sort of stalemate may be sufficient to loosen the grip of the complementary transference–countertransference relationship.

Containing

The concept of containment has a particular significance when a doctor is dealing psychodynamically with the personal level of clinical transactions, particularly those that have become complicated. It entails the capacity to be in touch with sometimes powerful or distressing feelings while at the same time resisting the impulse to give vent to them. Where these feelings come from may not always be obvious and the doctor may need to hold on to them for extended periods before this becomes any clearer. Containment has something in common with the familiar concept of masterly inactivity. For example, in a potentially threatening clinical situation, the doctor does not allow his or her anxiety to precipitate any hasty, ill-advised or unnecessary intervention. In this situation the doctor is helped by having all the relevant clinical data to hand and by his or her medical experience and training.

Containing feelings in a clinical transaction, where there are often no familiar guidelines, and where the feelings themselves may be the result of hidden or unconscious aspects of the doctor–patient interaction, often proves more difficult. The nature of the professional relationship itself places constraints on when, what, and how feelings are expressed and in most transactions these are kept within reasonable and appropriate bounds.

Complicated clinical transactions are often accompanied by feelings that are very intense and of a kind that recognisably fall outside the bounds of the professional relationship, or would do so if given expression. Containing them is important on two counts. First, it allows time for the doctor to search introspectively and attempt to understand what gives rise to such feelings. Second, the discipline of holding on to feelings helps to lessen the risk of simply retaliating or reacting to the patient. For instance, the interaction between doctor and patient may be enacting, via transference and countertransference, a theme of victim–victimiser. The patient may unconsciously project the sense of himself or herself as victim and thereby mobilise within the doctor a punitive or sadistic response (complementary countertransference). If the doctor can contain those projections and complementary responses, the possibility of a qualitatively different sort of engagement may emerge. For some patients it can be a powerful and novel experience to be responded to in a thoughtful way, and one of considerable therapeutic potential. By holding on to such feelings the doctor greatly enhances a patient's feeling of security. This can help to provide the basis for trust that may have been lacking in the relationships of his or her early life and that if developed will help to support the public interaction of the clinical transaction.

Containing, in the sense described above, may demand great effort and prove emotionally draining. Because of this it should be recognised as a positive intervention, even though there may be no manifest behavioural accompaniment. In itself it is likely to be a positive influence in a complicated transaction (or any transaction for that matter) and forms the necessary basis of empathy as well as of many useful interpretations.

Mr Osborne was twenty-two and a tough-looking character with chronic sinus problems. He did not help himself by smoking heavily and leading an irregular lifestyle, which involved drinking too much alcohol and 'clubbing' (attending night clubs) until the small hours each weekend. He had spent some of his teenage years living in institutional care. This followed the death of his mother from cancer. Quite unfairly, he seemed to be blamed for this by his father and stepmother. (Mr Osborne had been living alone with his mother when she died.)

Mr Osborne found great difficulty in asking for help of any kind and always presented in an aggressively demanding fashion. The doctor, who had known him for only two years (not during his teenage years), did not know any other members of the family, although she was aware of the above aspects of the history. Initially, she had felt somewhat intimidated by Mr Osborne's manner and behaviour and had not understood that part of the aggression he displayed was not so much personally directed as part of his more general difficulty with authority figures. He felt intensely humiliated and vulnerable when asking for help, as he was later able to confide. Initially, out of feelings of fear, the doctor had been quite dismissive of his demand for help with his sinuses and was caught up repeatedly in heated and unhelpful exchanges in which neither party appeared to hear the other's point of view. For her part, the doctor reiterated the need for him to make lifestyle changes. However, she felt uncomfortable with this state of affairs because she did not like the feeling that she was construed as being less helpful and understanding than she thought she actually was.

Having re-read the case-notes, which included some lengthy but informative social reports (also indicating that during adolescence Mr Osborne had been sexually abused while in care), the doctor felt more sympathetic towards him. Understanding that he had experienced little enough of a supportive family atmosphere in his formative years, she was more able to empathise, rather than take up a complementary position. This change in attitude was not reflected in any obvious behaviour on her part, save her not rising to the bait of her patient's aggressive demands. In 'doing nothing', but containing, she was surprised and relieved to observe that Mr Osborn's aggression subsided. Over the next year, he was in a sufficiently secure relationship with her to agree to specialist referral. He had resisted this option previously, it turned out, because of a clinically mild hospital phobia. He had associated all institutions with being in care, where any trust that might have been fostered had been betrayed.

Setting limits

At times, the doctor may need to set limits in the clinical transaction. Limits set may refer to the overt clinical goals of the transaction, in terms of what can and cannot be realistically expected. They may also refer to the behaviour of patient or doctor, in terms of what constitutes tolerable behaviour in the patient, or the lengths to which the doctor is able or prepared to go to help him or her. Setting limits, in an open and explicit way, may be unfamiliar territory for some doctors. It may involve confrontation and the risk of having to face a hostile or disappointed response from the patient, the prospect of which is an uncomfortable one, especially for those whose style is habitually non-confrontational. Anxiety on this account might be mitigated, however, in the knowledge that such hostility on the part of the patient may be a reflection of underlying depression or low self-steem. The doctor might further be encouraged by the thought that limit setting, implying as it does the need for accepting personal responsibility, self-discipline and clear boundaries, may be a therapeutic manoeuvre in itself. Patients' anxiety and consequent hostility is often fuelled by feeling ignorant and impotent about the illness, treatment or prognosis.

In clinical transactions where overt limit-setting becomes appropriate the patient is likely to have an impaired or fragile sense of self. For example, poor compliance with treatment might be an aspect of a patient's behaviour, betraying a self-destructive attitude, and this is why limits need to be set. The doctor in this situation, therefore, should proceed carefully and sensitively and a neutral rather than an overconcerned or confrontational approach is likely to be more fruitful. This may involve discussing the rationale for the approach and, if necessary, negotiating an alternative, acceptable avenue for self-destructive feelings. Even though initially such an approach might be greeted with further denial or disbelief, relief often ensues.

Obviously it is not possible to anticipate and describe all forms of unhelpful or subtly self-destructive behaviour that may complicate clinical transactions nor to indicate the appropriate response that should follow from the doctor. Each doctor–patient interaction is unique and, to an extent, the strategies deployed and negotiations carried out on the way to securing clinical goals will necessarily vary. However, the most usually problematic behaviours requiring limit-setting tend to centre on the following issues:

(1) too frequent attendance at the surgery, or too frequent telephone demands for advice or home visiting;
(2) inappropriate behaviour on the practice premises but outside the consulting room, such as verbal or physical aggression, or overtly amorous, disorderly or drunken behaviour (and including the bad behaviour of children);
(3) behaviour similar to that in (2) but within the consulting room;
(4) inappropriate demands or inappropriate goals of the clinical transaction, including both overt and covert goals.

In some instances, more than one or even all of the above may be present at the same time. On occasion, emergency measures may have to be taken by doctors and other practice staff, which may, for example, even entail calling in the police. Risk of physical injury or attack may be reduced by keeping reception staff behind effective safety barriers (see also Chapter 8) and having 'panic buttons' in surgeries. At other times matters can be dealt with less urgently and with less drama. Under suitable circumstances, the issue of setting limits can be discussed, by doctor and patient, together with the reasons for such an approach, and a contract can be negotiated between doctor or, in primary care settings, the practice as a whole and patient. The negotiating of treatment contracts may present many obstacles and pitfalls especially if it is an unfamiliar activity (see below).

Ms Parsons was a young single woman in her mid-twenties who had a serious drug misuse problem for which she had received much psychiatric and psychotherapeutic attention. This had included formal drug rehabilitation schemes. However, none of the treatments had secured lasting benefits. Ms Parsons seemed to be able to engineer admission to psychiatric hospital via a number of avenues: by presenting herself to the accident and emergency department; by presenting to the psychiatric hospital direct; or, more usually, by telephoning her primary care physician especially at night, when she was often particularly psychologically disturbed.

Ms Parsons was able to exert pressure on the various systems, by threatening or attempting suicide or by complaining of 'psychotic' symptoms, usually saying that she could hear the voice of the devil talking to her and commanding her to kill herself or commit some other atrocity. The psychiatric team who knew her best had diagnosed personality disorder in addition to drug misuse and believed that the 'psychotic' symptoms indeed might be authentic mental state phenomena (most likely related to drug withdrawal), which, however, were being presented with the conscious intention of gaining admission to hospital and escaping from inner tensions. The latter were contributed to by an unsatisfactory and unstable relationship with an aggressive and immature male partner.

Psychiatric advice to the primary care doctors involved (her indiscriminate nocturnal telephone conversations had involved all the doctors in the primary health care practice) was to stop responding to Ms Parson's distress calls by requesting psychiatric hospitalisation, even though it was acknowledged there was a real risk that she might kill herself or harm others. This advice was reinforced through discussion with all of the medical staff involved and with Ms Parson's social worker and probation officer.

None of the professionals involved with Ms Parsons was entirely happy with the plan, even though this had been mutually agreed. What had emerged at discussion was a clear agreement that the current situation was deteriorating, as evidenced by escalating self-injurious behaviour and more frequent telephone calls. It was agreed therefore that a change in clinical management was called for, since Ms Parsons herself continuing to exert control over the available caring services was unhelpful.

It was decided that limits would be set with regard to what was an acceptable caring response on the part of the professionals involved. Ms Parsons, who was involved in the discussion (although only after the professionals had met and agreed the plan) was reluctant to accept the idea that psychiatric in-patient treatment would not be available and that instead she would have to make a choice of whether or not to use the weekly sessions that were offered by her social worker and psychiatrist together. She was told that the primary care doctors would not offer any psychological support beyond being courteous to her on the telephone nor would they make requests for her to be hospitalised. She would simply be directed by them, if crises arose, to attend the weekly sessions.

The above hard-won agreement and management plan were repeatedly tested by Ms Parsons. Sometimes the professionals were able to withstand her attempts to control and manipulate but at other times they were not and she would be admitted to hospital (albeit briefly). The primary care doctors, from time to time, attempted to pressure the psychiatric team into accepting total responsibility for the treatment of Ms Parsons and asked for her to be admitted as a long-term psychiatric patient. Heated exchanges occurred between primary and secondary care doctors, which necessitated further meetings of all professionals concerned in the management of the case. On the basis of one such meeting it was agreed to persevere with the previously agreed plan but to instigate three-monthly meetings of all concerned in order to review the situation. This plan appeared to help. Certainly the primary and secondary care doctor were better able to see one another's points of view and as a result the former felt less hostile to what they perceived was a lack of psychiatric support. Previously, the primary care doctors had felt let down by the secondary level of care in not providing in-patient admission as a response to Ms Parson's frequent crises in spite of being party to the management strategy.

The above plan in fact continued for three years, at the end of which time Ms Parsons had not been an in-patient in a psychiatric ward for more than a year. She admitted that she felt more in control of her own life. She had also managed to break from her partner, which she viewed as a positive development. Her relationship with her family, which had previously been poor, had improved. She remained, however, highly dependent upon her weekly sessions with the psychiatrist and social worker and there was no plan to discontinue these, at least for the foreseeable future. The professionals involved in the case also felt some degree of pride and satisfaction in having been able to facilitate clinical gains through the process of limit-setting. They viewed their initial disquiet and difficulty with maintaining the limits as almost a necessary phase of the treatment without which they would not have been able to have collaborated so closely and cohesively to provide a clinical environment that did not reinforce unhealthy behaviour but rather facilitated a more mature use of the caring services available.

Negotiating treatment contracts

When elucidation, education and interpretation have failed to unlock a complicated clinical transaction and the doctor needs to set limits, the use of a treatment contract should be considered. In such a situation the implicit contract between doctor and patient, based on their respective social roles, is no longer sufficient to sustain the clinical transaction. The renegotiation of an explicit treatment contract is thus required. This serves to bolster the public level of the doctor–patient interaction by making explicit the conditions required for doctor and patient to continue their transaction. It reinforces what are to be considered the legitimate goals of the transaction and indicates those that are not. The consequences of inappropriate goal-seeking behaviour on the part of the patient are made clear and a treatment contract builds into the situation what can be expected of the doctor by clarifying what he or she will and will not do or tolerate.

The main point of a treatment contract is to set limits on the patient's behaviour. The contract serves this purpose in a number of ways (Miller, 1989) by:

(1) assisting the patient's self control;
(2) minimising the patient's feelings of rejection (by specifying limits in advance rather than imposing them in the heat of an angry exchange);
(3) decreasing an oppositional stance, inviting the patient to accept the responsibility and risks of complying with treatment;
(4) defusing primitive idealisation or denigration of the doctor, likely when immature defence mechanisms are operating (see Chapter 4).

The use of a treatment contract is particularly helpful where the prominent deployment of immature defence mechanisms has led to the transaction becoming complicated. The approach can be used regardless of the presenting complaint or illness and irrespective of the specific diagnosis and treatment details. Nor need it imply who has caused the complication. After all, transactions become complicated as a result of an interaction between doctor and patient and it is not always possible, or even necessary, to decide whose immature defences may have been erected first!

The contract will focus upon, specifically, departures from appropriate help-seeking behaviour and attitudes and the doctor will have to carefully monitor both public and personal levels of the interaction. Because it is not always clear what his or her own contribution to any complication might be, it may pay the doctor to discuss complicated clinical transactions, and any treatment contracts being considered, within a group of interested colleagues (see Chapter 8). It is likely anyway, that to be successful in a primary care setting, a treatment contact will need the co-operation of other doctors or practice staff even if they are not directly involved. Otherwise doctors or other staff may be set against one another (as in the earlier example) or, acting in ignorance, breach the bounds of the contract.

Mrs Arkwright, at seventy, was bedridden due to the sequelae of longstanding osteoporosis. She inhabited a bed in the living-room of the home she shared with her aging and mildly dementing husband and her forty-four year old daughter, Stella. The district nurses attended daily and her family doctor visited once per month. In spite of her physical state, Mrs Arkwright was in full command of her other faculties and also had a sharp tongue.

Problems of clinical management arose on two counts. Mrs Arkwright was constantly demanding of the nurses and equally constant in her criticism of them. Not only could they do very little right, but she continuously complained to them about the doctor, whom she believed did not visit her often enough. When the doctor did visit, however, she became a model patient, with effusive expressions of gratitude and appreciation for the doctor's time and attention.

It emerged that the daughter, Stella, under the influence of alcohol, was with increasing frequency violent to both parents. Although by far the strongest physically of the three, at times she was in fact dominated by her mother. So serious did matters become that Mrs Arkwright repeatedly threatened to have Stella forcibly evicted from the home and with this endeavour she tried to enlist the support of the nurses involved with her. She would always relent, however, short of the point at which any action would be taken saying that for herself and her husband to lose their daughter would break the husband's heart. Nevertheless, she would continue her threats again, within a short period, and exhort the nurses and doctor to voice similar threats. She expressed the belief to the nurses that the doctor had the power not only to stop Stella being violent but also to organise the latter's eviction if he so chose. The doctor had in fact seen Stella on her own account, for alcohol-related physical problems. She had confessed to her aggressive behaviour towards her parents and had appeared contrite, promising to desist. However, she also requested advice on how she might organise residential care for her parents!

The violence escalated and the situation became progressively more difficult to manage. Finally, the nurses organised: first, a meeting of all the carers who were involved with the family in order to discuss how best to manage the situation; second, a meeting jointly between those carers and the three members of the family. At the second meeting, it was made clear to Mrs Arkwright that the doctor did not have any relevant authority to remove Stella from the parental home against her will and that entreaties to any of the caring professionals regarding this matter would be ignored. However, at the same time Mrs Arkwright was given information about whom it would be appropriate to contact for legal advice on the matter. (Thus limits were set on what was appropriate public domain business.) It was made clear to Stella that the only role for staff in respect of herself was to help her with obtaining appropriate psychological treatment for her alcohol dependence. Furthermore, the doctor and nurses (having discussed the strategy beforehand) stated that they would continue only to provide care in respect of Mrs Arkwright's physical complaints and in respect of Stella's alcohol-related problems. The doctor indicated, however, that he was prepared to increase the frequency of his visits (to fortnightly) but that these would be strictly time-limited. Following discussion, the Arkwrights agreed to the 'contract', not without reluctance.

This contract did not completely solve the problems of the Arkwright family and their carers. However, it did enhance the team spirit of the professionals involved and, in particular, helped the nurses to cope with the constant complaining about matters outside their control. The doctor's increased visiting also helped to provide support to the nursing staff. Mrs Arkwright discontinued her complaints about the doctor and even though Stella did not accept help for her alcohol problem, and she continued to drink excessively on occasions, the violence disappeared. Mrs Arkwright did continue to voice complaints about Stella but without her previous venom.

Ideally, in order to be effective, a treatment contract must be mutually agreed by all likely to be involved, not just doctor and patient. Sometimes, other family members will have to be party to the contract, especially in the case of children or adolescents. Achievable goals and the strategies to achieve them should be clearly specified and include the responsibilities of both the doctor and patient, making clear what the doctor can and cannot be expected to provide or tolerate. That having been said, the contract should aim to set a minimum number of conditions, but sufficient to safeguard the patient and the treatment.

Resort to treatment contracts should only take place when the limits of the normal transactions have been repeatedly or dangerously breached, as in the case of the Arkwrights. Patients involved often have poor self-control and a limited capacity to tolerate frustration and anxiety. The contract may therefore be precarious, especially as it may demand that patients forego their usual means of managing intolerable feelings. The availability of the doctor should be specified in advance, as far as is possible, and alternative strategies prepared and agreed for times when he or she is not available. Written treatment contracts may carry extra weight when signed by all parties. They can be of value, for example, in the management of those seeking help for drug and alcohol addiction.

Successful operation of the contract entails the use of positive reinforcement and encouragement when conditions are met and goals attained. If the contract is generated at a time when doctor or patient are in the grip of hostile or punitive feelings towards one another, such operation is unlikely to develop. Once established, however, any treatment contact should be strictly enforced, although allowing for reasonable, negotiated modifications (Miller, 1989).

Risks to the treatment contract occur when these guidelines are not followed. Common errors therefore include:

(1) punitive or rejecting use of contracts, which have been made in the heat of the moment, when doctor and patient are feeling hostile towards one another;
(2) infantilisation of the patient through the imposition of a one-sided, non-negotiable contract with too many conditions;
(3) removing the only defences against intolerable feelings that the patient knows, without offering alternatives;

(4) allowing any outside professionals involved to specify unrealistic treatment conditions (see below).

Integrating treatment approaches

The possibility arises, where more than one professional or agency is involved in treating a patient, as in the example of Ms Parsons, that approaches to treatment may conflict (representing adverse influences arising out of conflicting goals of different systems), rather than being facilitatory or synergistic. Those involved may be oblivious to inherent contradictions, and patients, should they recognise such contradictions, may be too timid or annoyed to point them out. As discussed in earlier chapters, patients with immature personalities and associated chronic problems with regulating self-esteem may have difficulty in performing the sick role appropriately. When faced with the unspoken and unacknowledged incompatibility of treatment approaches, such patients may act to maintain or exacerbate the conflictual situation by following no single treatment exactly. In some instances the efforts of other professionals will be idealised or denigrated, while the doctor's own efforts are experienced in the opposite mode. The doctor may then be drawn into a complementary countertransference or end up siding with the patient against the other professional (as in the case of Mrs Jones with the irritable bowel and the enamoured doctor, in Chapter 6).

It is quite possible that the goals or requirements of different treatment approaches are mutually exclusive, for example one displaying tolerance of deviant behaviour (such as self-mutilation or parasuicidal acts), while the other sets clearly defined limits, specifying the negative consequences should these be transgressed. Particularly problematic may be the period of transfer or transition from an episode of in-patient treatment to out-patient, day care or community-based treatment. This may involve different key personnel or discharge to the doctor's sole care. Case conferences, gathering together all those concerned and involved with the treatment, can be extremely useful in identifying any differences in treatment approach. These can then be discussed and resolved and a co-ordinated approach decided. In this context the use of treatment contracts may have much to commend it. In some instances failure of professionals to resolve their conflicting treatment approaches can have serious consequences for the patient. In such situations, it is particularly important for the doctors involved in any clinical transactions with the patient to be sensitive to the influence of external systems. The example below demonstrates how even apparently minor discrepancies in treatment approach can produce deleterious effects.

Mr Simmonds presented to his doctor with a complaint of depressed mood. His wife was slowly dying from an inoperable ovarian cancer and he became preoccupied by his seven year old son's reaction to his wife's illness. The son had become enuretic and teachers had commented that his behaviour at school, having been previously unremarkable, had become aggressive. Mr Simmonds asked for advice on how best he might deal with the situation and, specifically, what and how much he should tell his son about the mother's illness and impending death. Perhaps mistakenly, Mr Simmonds asked the same question of both the primary and secondary care doctors. The former advocated his spending more time with the son and answering questions simply without evasion. The latter informed Mr Simmonds that his son could not possibly understand the complexities of the situation and should not be burdened with them.

Mr Simmonds brooded on this conflicting advice, although he believed both advisers had been well intentioned. His own depression prevented him from challenging the advice or mentioning the conflict, the burden of which he was left to shoulder. After his wife died, his son's behaviour continued to deteriorate at school and he was eventually referred to an educational psychologist and subsequently to a child psychiatrist. Mr Simmonds felt himself to blame for his son's difficulties. The overall effect was to complicate his own grieving process for his wife. It was his continuing depression, some two years after his wife's death, which brought him again to his doctor, when the above history emerged.

This example demonstrates how an apparently incidental detail involving the imparting of conflictual advice had serious ramifications. In this instance, this did not so much contribute to Mr Simmonds' depression as to his delayed presentation to his doctor, to say nothing of the effect on his son.

Interviewing other parties

In primary care settings the doctor's task in integrating different treatment approaches may be analogous to that of the patient who has to resolve issues arising from the conflicting influences of his or her family and social network (systemic influences). Advice from family members about illness and its treatment may conflict with the doctor's advice and the effect on the patient may be identical with the situation where professional advice is contradictory. It may be sufficient to take an educative approach, making the patient aware, and allowing discussion, of conflicting influences. When this proves ineffective it can be helpful and enlightening to interview others involved, usually the patient's partner or family. In the field of primary care medicine, the opportunity to gather useful information often arises coincidentally when other members of the family attend on their own account. However, such attendances may not be entirely coincidental and may reflect an inappropriate level of involvement and concern of a family with each other's problems. Managing confidentiality and other boundary issues can prove a delicate task but often relevant strands of information can be woven together from such encounters, which throw light upon management difficulties. More formal interviews can be arranged where appropriate, if those involved are agreeable. Co-operation of family or partner may be necessary in certain instances where treatment contracts are being considered.

The doctor treating Mrs North (Chapter 1) for her agoraphobia believed that it was important for the patient's daughter to be interviewed, with her mother, since she had played such an important role initially in supporting mother after the episode of pericarditis as well as then, unwittingly, in precipitating the agoraphobia itself. An explanation of the complexities of the situation not only gave the treatment itself a greater chance of success but the daughter almost certainly was helped to avoid feeling inappropriately guilty at her own role in the promotion of mother's psychological condition.

Terminating treatment

Often the ending of a consultation or treatment episode receives less attention than do the diagnostic and active treatment phases. This may pose few or no problems in many instances and the clinical transaction proceeds smoothly and is completed satisfactorily – a straightforward clinical transaction. However, this is by no means always the case and the conclusion of a transaction may be marred by many factors, including the persistence of residual symptoms, the absence of effective treatment or the inevitable worsening of a chronic condition. Concluding a treatment episode may become problematic if a patient's psychosocial circumstances change in such a way that he or she finds giving up the sick role difficult or unattractive. In other instances a patient (or doctor) may, for quite personal reasons, have difficulty with endings in general. This difficulty may be irrespective of the quality of the transaction up to that point. Inappropriate difficulty with endings is more likely to be the product of insecure attachments or of particular styles of doctor–patient interaction, especially those where doctor or patient prominently display immature defence mechanisms, which deny, displace or minimise any relevant emotional aspects.

For many patients, the changes associated with endings are emotionally difficult because they bring with them echoes of past losses or endings that have been only incompletely accepted. Unresolved grief is a common and obvious example. Sometimes patients and doctors are brought into prolonged and intimate contact because of the nature of a given illness or transaction. The end of the treatment episode may then conjure up feelings, in the present, that are inappropriate in their range or intensity. This is because they also derive from past losses or endings. Discharge from a prolonged period of hospitalisation can sometimes prove to be an event from which the patient never fully recovers, emotionally or psychologically, despite apparent physical cure. Hospitalisation on account of psychiatric disorder may be particularly likely to result in difficulty readjusting to the demands of everyday life. It may be beneficial, therefore, to acknowledge and discuss the difficulties inherent in recovery from hospitalisation, as well as from the problems caused by the illness itself.

In such situations, and with certain patients who may be particularly sensitised to issues concerning loss or separation, the doctor must take care that he or she avoids inadvertently contributing to these problems, rather than relieving them. A common example, in primary care settings, is the situation where a doctor has struggled to help a depressed or anxious patient in the course of several appointments over many weeks. Finally, acknowledging that little progress is being made, the doctor might suggest referral for psychiatric or psychological help. If this entails the abrupt cessation of appointments with the doctor, the patient may feel a sense of loss or rejection that can actually exacerbate the condition itself.

A poignant example is the case of Miss Hallam, a successful single woman, who gave up a full-time career to nurse her aging and widowed mother, with whom she lived. Mrs Hallam had an inoperable malignancy and, often in pain, grew weaker. Her doctor, who had been the one to make the diagnosis, attended with increasing frequency as time wore on and towards the end visited daily, sometimes more than once. He admired the efficiency and tenderness with which

Miss Hallam nursed her mother and he got on well with her. When Mrs Hallam died he was able to attend promptly and lend some immediate comfort to her daughter. But after that his visits stopped. Some time later Miss Hallam attended surgery looking worn out and upset. She appeared hostile and soon it became clear that she felt angry with the doctor for not diagnosing her mother's cancer in time for something to be done. The doctor sympathetically tried to answer questions and explained that by the time the cancer had become symptomatic it had already been incurable. He identified her continuing grief and suggested she see a counsellor. It emerged later, through further meetings with Miss Hallam and discussion with the counsellor, that some of Miss Hallam's anger and grief arose not only from the loss of her mother but also from the abrupt loss of contact with the doctor. She had experienced this as an abandonment and it had awoken in her the pain of the loss many years earlier of her father, to whom she had been particularly close (more so than to her mother). She had not been able to grieve this loss fully since at the time she had felt her mother's loss of her husband to be the more important loss and had rallied behind her offering emotional support. With counselling, Miss Hallam's grief subsided but thereafter, on the rare occasions she needed to see a doctor, she chose to see one of the other doctors in the practice.

Regardless of the length of treatment, and even in the case of an individual encounter, it pays the doctor to attend carefully to endings. Much obviously depends on the personal qualities that the doctor brings to the relationships with his or her patients. Wherever possible, in clinical transactions spanning more than one consultation, endings should be planned or negotiated together with the patient. In this way the straightforward clinical transaction can be upheld and the patient may not need to complicate it, for example by inappropriately presenting further complaints just before the end in order to avoid the stress of the ending itself. An extra session or a longer appointment to deal with the leaving may be beneficial in the long run, assuming that such time is spent dealing with termination issues. Time taken to ventilate feelings of sadness or anger at the end of treatment may avoid further traumatising a vulnerable patient with yet more unresolved feelings associated with loss. This may be especially true where residual symptoms persist, or the illness is chronic or incurable. Attending to the personal domain in this way increases the likelihood that future clinical transactions will be straightforward.

Using medication

The prescribing and taking of medication, often apparently straightforward activities and part of the public domain, can represent behaviours that complicate the clinical transaction. Within the bounds of the straightforward clinical transaction the diagnosis will determine whether or not the doctor prescribes a given drug. Thus, for the most part, the prescribing, dispensing and taking of medication is carried on straightforwardly and represents stable public domain activity. However, there are psychodynamic factors that increase the likelihood of either over- or under-medicating patients, potentially complicating the clinical transaction (Miller, 1989).

Medication can represent a substitute gratification for unmet interpersonal needs (Havers, 1968) with the attendant risks, in some situations, of dependence and overdose. Under certain conditions, medication can be construed as rewarding infantile or otherwise immature behaviour and therefore encouraging more of the same (Friedman, 1969). Medication can be used creatively, as if a substitute for the destructive alternatives (Green *et al.*, 1988), with the medication representing, in some sense, healthy dependency on the doctor (Adelman, 1983). The prescription of medication may represent the prescription of authority. Where patients have problems with authority figures, the doctor may be tempted to become authoritarian, adopting a complementary role to the correspondingly weak and helpless patient. A master–slave dynamic may be enacted in this way. Medication can usefully become a forum for negotiation, if not over the precise drug, then over the working out of a convenient and practical dosage schedule. The patient is thus encouraged to take responsibility for the management of his or her own condition in partnership with the doctor (Green *et al.*, 1988). The doctor may resort to medicating as a signal that his or her own personal resources are used up, or to alleviate anxiety, or to express anger (which may be a particular risk when dealing with patients whose strong emotions prove difficult to contain – often those with immature personalities). The fact that medication may be used as a non-verbal way of controlling feelings may contradict what, under some circumstances, are the therapeutic goals of teaching patients to manage feelings with words (Graff and Mallin, 1967).

Conclusions

It is not possible for the doctor to know in advance the best approach to adopt in dealing with a complicated clinical transaction. What is most important is to have an understanding of the range of influences that may exert a complicating effect. The doctor's first task, therefore, is to try to avoid contributing to further complication by inadvertent or automatic responses, ranging from non-verbal behaviour to inappropriate investigation, treatment or secondary referral. Transient and minor departures from the straightforward clinical transaction are of no clinical significance and require no action or change in the doctor's usual style.

Sometimes, in the face of a complicated clinical transaction, the doctor does not have to do anything differently except to provide more time for explanation, reassurance or advice. Especially when treatment outcome is known to be unsatisfactory or in some way response to treatment is incomplete, attention to the endings of a treatment episode is important, especially to allow the patient space to ventilate attendant negative feelings. Although difficult at the time, ensuring that sufficient time has been put aside for the task may yield long-term benefits in terms of the straightforwardness of future clinical transactions.

Complication may set in at any stage of the clinical transaction and, to an extent, the issues involved at different stages vary, as do the responses required of the doctor in dealing with them. Elucidating and encouraging the patient to divulge information will be strategies that tend to be deployed earlier. Interpretation and confrontation cannot usually be successfully used early on in a clinical transaction. A certain amount of prior contact and, ideally, a reasonably empathic earlier relationship enhances the success of such strategies. Where ventilation of feelings, obtaining more information and education have failed to return a complicated clinical transaction to the straightforward, interpretation may be the next step. Confrontation and limit-setting will tend to be later strategies.

Sometimes, however, confrontation and limit-setting are earlier activities because of gross and obvious departures from the straightforward clinical transaction. Such interventions should not be seen as signs of failure, since in some clinical situations the only way to facilitate the straightforward clinical transaction is via the use of such techniques. Setting limits on a patient's negative behaviour is problematic, especially when the patient does not have an alternative response to deploy. A carefully negotiated treatment contract may therefore be useful. The pitfalls identified above, however, need to be studiously avoided. Careful attention should also be given to the manner in which doctor and patient address the endings of clinical transactions, particularly when they have been complicated or involved prolonged or serious illness.

8

Implications for the clinical setting

Introduction

Potentially, the doctor–patient interaction, being an open system, is crucially affected by its immediate physical, emotional and social environment. In this chapter, aspects of the structure and organisation of the wider clinical setting are examined, as they may influence the clinical transaction so as to increase the risk of complication. Certain features of clinics are shared by both primary care and hospital-based out-patient settings. However, issues of size and scale are important and not all the aspects considered apply equally to each setting. Clinical transactions, especially complicated ones, influence the function of the supra-system of the clinic. Thus, the relationship between clinical transaction and the wider clinical context is interactive. Ways in which this interaction can be manifest are examined. Organisational structures that can reduce the potential for complicated transactions are described.

The physical setting

The physical setting of clinics forms part of the 'frame' in which the clinical transaction unfolds and should be acknowledged as being part of the therapist's communication with the patient (Langs, 1978). The setting not only communicates something attributable to the particular doctors who work there but it also conveys something about the system of health care as a whole, of which the clinic is only a part or subsystem. This potentially powerful form of non-verbal communication therefore makes its statement and has its effect at both public and personal levels.

The physical aspects of a clinical setting include the buildings and their location, the external and internal decoration, and the arrangements for reception, waiting areas, consulting and treatment rooms. Before the

128

patient ever speaks to a member of the clinic staff, the first elements of the process that becomes the clinical transaction have begun. It is, therefore, of some importance that the communication made by the physical setting is what is intended or, at least, that some assessment is made of its potential or likely effect.

The physical setting should both permit and facilitate the clinical transactions that are pursued within its bounds. To this end buildings must fulfil public domain criteria necessary in order to function as intended. They must be, for example, clean and safe, accessible and equipped for the tasks to be carried on within. If they are not adequate, then meeting the conditions for a straightforward clinical transaction may be already jeopardised before doctor and patient have even met. But the physical setting also conveys an impression to its users about the manner in which it fulfils the functions it serves.

To the extent that the architecture or decor approach the limits of what is acceptable, the communication to the patient becomes more and more one that operates at the personal level. Beyond the limits of acceptability it is liable to evoke overt personal reactions, negative or positive, which may be strong enough to influence the interaction with the non-clinical staff and doctors (or other clinicians). An example of this was the use of vibrant primary colours in the internal decoration of a new primary care clinic, which provoked comments of reproach or affront from patients as they entered the consulting room. These had to be acknowledged in one way or another by the doctor.

A spectrum of possible communications a setting might convey can be imagined by considering the likely effect on patients of the waiting area seating arrangements illustrated in Figure 8.1.

Anything about the physical setting that deviates from a neutral 'appropriateness', be it music playing in the waiting area, the uniforms of the reception staff, or the seating arrangements in the consulting rooms, is likely to communicate something to patients at a personal level. In some circumstances this may be sufficient to contribute importantly to later complications in the clinical transaction. In this respect any such architectural deviations are analogous to departures from the doctor's usual style, behaviour, thoughts and feelings during the clinical transaction. This is not to say that deviations from emotionally or aesthetically neutral appropriateness should never happen but rather that the potential they have to communicate something significant to patients (which might also increase the risk of complicating the clinical transactions) should be anticipated.

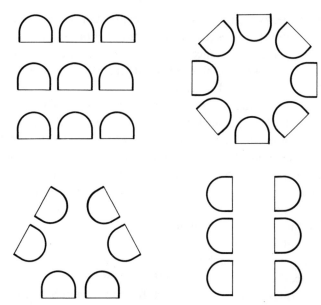

Figure 8.1. Different seating arrangements in a waiting area may convey something significant about the clinic to those waiting.

Change to an established physical setting is particularly likely to communicate something that may affect the transaction. Seating arrangements are well known to have an effect on consulting behaviour (see Pietroni, 1976). As an example, one doctor changed the seating arrangement in his consulting room so that instead of facing the patient across the corner of his desk he sat virtually knee to knee with the patient. For a while the implicit change in the interpersonal boundaries between doctor and patient had quite a disturbing effect on the doctor. That this was also true of some of the longstanding patients was demonstrated by more than one coming into the room and moving the chair back to its former position. Another doctor in the clinic, who had adopted a similar seating arrangement, and had become quite used to it, was surprised at the emotional impact made on her when a disabled patient was wheeled in and placed opposite her, with the desk between them.

At the personal level, an individual patient's reactions to the physical setting of a clinic will depend on aspects of his or her personality and personal life experience. The foundations of such individual reactions may well be, in large part, outside conscious awareness. At the public level, in serving its social function, the practice must satisfy certain public criteria, as mentioned above. To the extent that it meets or fails to meet these criteria, and the extent to which it deviates from an architectural norm, it may be construed by patients in terms of the overall quality of care being offered.

Management of anxiety

One of the functions of the clinic system is to contain anxiety that arises out of, and relates to, issues of intimacy, incapacity and death and hence in relation to illness and its treatment (Obholzer, 1989). The containment of emotions and feelings was discussed in Chapter 7 in terms of its importance for the interaction of doctor and patient (as individuals) within the clinical transaction. In this context, it serves to emphasise the importance of the physical setting insofar as its design, for instance, should be welcoming and reassuring, rather than jarring or exciting.

The physical setting of a clinic should, therefore, reflect its function of containing the anxiety of illness and death. However, in performing this function, the setting will also reflect something of the needs of those who work there and whose professional responsibility is to maintain composure and provide comfort in the face of the demands and threats of illness. Aspects of the physical setting may reflect unconscious as well as conscious needs of staff to distance or defend themselves from those demands and anxieties. In most clinics, patients and staff are unambiguously separated by the physical structure of the building, for example by the receptionist's hatch (and also, perhaps, by the use of a uniform for the staff). In many clinics in primary care, the doctors' common room, if there is one, is as far from the patients' waiting area as it is physically possible to be within the building. As well as there being sensible and logistic reasons for this, there may be an unconscious defensive aspect to such siting, which, in some circumstances, may reflect an attitude toward the patient as enemy and which may also contribute to the propensity to stigmatically label certain patients.

Clinic organisation

The organisation of a clinic both affects, and less obviously is affected by, the clinical transaction. Clinical transactions in general demand certain organisational structures and processes to sustain them. These structures must serve the function of bringing together doctor and patient to address the practical tasks of health care in a private and confidential setting. In this way the clinic organisation and clinical transaction interact, each with the potential to influence the other.

The organisational structure of a clinic consists of many elements but especially those relatively fixed aspects considered necessary to allow the clinic to function. These include the kind and number of employed and attached staff, the doctors themselves, appointment systems, information systems, hours of business, on-call arrangement, financial systems, and systems of internal and external communication. Management consists of those processes that create, maintain, and develop the organisation. The working of the clinic obviously involves myriad personal interactions both at the organisational level and the management level. These interactions are pursued at both public and personal levels, and, to the extent that they are directed towards a goal, i.e. are transactions, they can be straightforward or complicated.

During his or her passage to the clinical transaction itself, the patient negotiates, primarily, with the organisational structure of the clinic. As with the physical setting, the organisational structure communicates something to the patient. Those aspects of clinic organisation of most immediate and obvious relevance are the appointment system and reception. The first of these, while operated by people, is in itself impersonal. The patient cannot be said to enter into a transaction with an appointment system and yet he or she will infer many things about the wider practice or hospital from it. The receptionists are often the first people in the clinic to interact with patients. Both these systems, therefore, may have effects on the patient that can subsequently influence the clinical transaction.

The appointment system

Much has been written about appointment systems in primary care settings, for example, about appointment length, duration of clinic, time of day and appointment versus open surgeries (Arber and Sawyer, 1982; Wilson, 1991). Such aspects have been evaluated in terms of the effects they have on the patient and the doctor and some systems are considered better than others. At the public level, an appointment system simultaneously allows and regulates access to the doctor. Ideally, it helps doctor and patient organise their time so that patients are not kept waiting overlong or unpredictably or doctors are not overwhelmed and have time to attend to other medical (or non-medical) tasks. Problems obviously arise for patients, receptionists and doctors, when demand for appointments outstrips supply. This is a common problem and can be an arena in which many a battle is fought. Such problems have many causes that are often not easily rectified.

In fulfilling, or failing to fulfil, these functions, an appointment system is capable of communicating many things at the personal level, some of which may hold inherent contradictions. On the one hand, an appointment may represent a symbolic token and guarantee of the forthcoming meeting with the doctor but, on the other hand, it sets limits to this meeting. It implies, in fact, both a meeting and a parting.

Patients may have ambivalent or mixed feelings about doctors, or indeed medicine in general, but at some level the meeting with the doctor holds some hope, or fear, as well as public domain expectations to be correctly diagnosed and appropriately treated. Often this will include a wish for an explanation of symptoms and diagnosis and, in addition, relief from both mental and physical suffering. At a deeper level, symptoms, or simply the idea of visiting the doctor, may have stirred profound anxieties about intimacy, incapacity or death itself, even if these remain unacknowledged. The knowledge that an appointment has been made can function to contain a patient's anxiety while he or she is waiting to see the doctor or it may hang over him or her like a portent of doom; it may be something of each.

An appointment indicates that the patient has only limited access to the doctor and implies that the doctor has other patients to see. These imposed limits bolster the doctor's capacity to tolerate and contain the patient's projected anxieties to which he or she is exposed, and which, operating mostly at an unconscious level, may awaken primitive anxieties of his or her own.

At the public level, the conflicting functions of the appointment are reflected within the roles of doctor and patient. The doctor will endeavour to meet the patient's needs but only if the patient presents these in manageable amounts. On the personal level, the patient has the satisfaction of having the doctor to himself or herself but only for a limited time. In one respect the patient is unique and special, in another just one of many. Patients respond to the constraints of the appointment in different ways. Some may be acutely aware of the doctor's time; some only too eager to be in and out; others may have covert or unconscious goals, which lead them to ignore the limits imposed by the appointment for one reason or another. As discussed in the last chapter, some may have special difficulties with endings. Doctors, for their part, may be more or less tolerant of the demand of the patient to control the time taken. The appointment system will reflect these tensions by allocating lengths of time that are more or less generous and, in this way, it represents something of the attitude of the clinic system, as a whole, to its patients.

Obviously appointment lengths and clinic times, and other aspects of the clinical setting for that matter, are also constrained by factors such as finance or staffing, including absences of staff due to holidays or sickness. Once again, the way in which a clinic deals with such obstacles or constraints will be interpreted by patients, at the personal level, as a communication of the quality of caring offered, not only by the clinic but by the health care system as a whole. Also reflected will be something of the doctor's personal attitude to his or her patient and how he or she handles the tension between the perceived pressure to meet patients' needs and demands and the need to control or restrict them. Therefore what appear to be relatively mundane problems concerning appointment systems may need to be examined with a rigour and sensitivity analogous to those pertaining to the clinical transaction.

Reception

The physical setting and the appointment system, while communicating something to the patient about the clinic, do not permit a dialogue. Any communication from the patient, concerning these aspects of the clinic, has to wait until human contact is made. The first person the patient speaks to, over the counter, through the hatch or on the telephone, is likely to be the receptionist. At this point begins the complex process of interpersonal transactions that is to be pursued at public and personal levels. Reception staff may have little training and are often taken for granted (Copeman and Zwanenberg, 1988). Traditionally they have a poor public image as far as patient opinion is concerned (Arber and Sawyer, 1985).

Patient and receptionist engage in a transaction (in the sense of interacting to negotiate a goal), which may be straightforward or complicated. A major role receptionists perform within the clinic entails that they act as intermediaries between the patient and the purveyors of health care in the practice, i.e. the doctors, nurses and any other attached clinical staff. The receptionist is involved in a relationship with both the doctor (or other clinicians) and the patient. Therefore, the receptionist's relationship with the patient is implicitly triangular (Figure 8.2). It comprises one actual transaction (bounded by the continuous lines in Figure 8.2), between the receptionist and the patient, and two that are implicit (bounded by the broken lines), between patient and clinician, and receptionist and clinician, respectively.

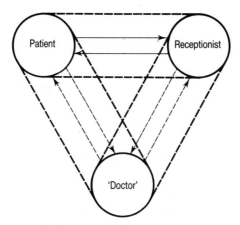

Figure 8.2. The transaction between patient and receptionist may be influenced by their transactions (real or imagined) with the doctor or provider of health care. The bold lines indicate the boundaries of the systems; the lines with arrows denote interactions.

The doctor (or other clinical member of the primary or secondary health care team) may be known to the patient or else a stranger. If the latter, the patient may have in mind a stereotypical doctor or other professional, having the qualities, skills and functions of his or her role, but coloured by the patient's prior experience of doctors and other carers or figures of authority from the past. If the former, often the case in primary care settings, the patient has in mind a particular doctor with known personal attributes. In this situation the patient will already be in a relationship based on his or her previous experience of that individual. Aspects of that existing relationship may influence the interaction with the receptionist. In this respect, a receptionist may relate that a patient has been angry or abusive (especially when appointments are scarce), when immediately afterwards the same patient has been a model of compliance and respect in the presence of the doctor. In at least some of such instances the receptionist may have become the receptacle of the patient's dissatisfaction with a particular doctor, or, perhaps, with the clinic or health service as a whole. Although such anger may be fully justified, at another level it should be remembered that a perceived failure of care may also have its roots in other contexts of the patient's life, past or present. Also, it may reflect the patient's incapacity to tolerate an ordinary amount of frustration that, as a consequence, is dealt with via the unconscious use of immature defence mechanisms, resulting in, for example, intense anger, which is denied in one setting and displaced to another.

Patient and receptionist may be, simultaneously, members of the overlapping systems (for example, families or social class), which bring to bear influences capable of distorting the patient–receptionist transaction even further. Distortions in the patient–receptionist transaction can be carried over into the clinical transaction with the doctor. If sufficiently pronounced, they can become complicating factors in this transaction (i.e. an adverse systemic influence).

Mrs Browne, who had been unable to arrange a suitable appointment to see her regular doctor, decided to go to the surgery, taking the chance that an appointment could be made there and then. When this did not take place and she was seen subsequently (in fact, the next day) by the doctor, she complained bitterly about the rudeness and unhelpfulness of the receptionist with whom she had negotiated the consultation. The doctor offered some placatory remarks but, after a few minutes of the consultation, Mrs Browne, obviously distressed, blurted out that she was too upset to continue and hastily left.

The blame or responsibility for a situation such as this cannot, of course, solely be placed at the receptionist's door as it is likely to be also a reflection of the receptionist's relationship with the doctor and the overall clinic policy towards appointments and, of course, factors in the patient need to be taken into account. However, the receptionist's transaction with Mrs Browne was complicated, even though the likely cause, in this instance, was an adverse systemic influence arising out of clinic policy, which was not to allow appointments to be made once a clinic had begun.

If certain problems, or problems with certain patients, happen recurrently, it can be worth while examining all three possible transactions in the patient–receptionist–doctor triangle using the transaction window. Such an analysis can be extended to other complicated (non-clinical) transactions that emerge from time to time within a given clinic or wider healthcare setting and be incorporated into the overall management systems.

Clinic management

Successful clinic management rests ultimately on processes that harness and harmonise the interactions of the people involved. In practice, not all of these will be harmonious but, ideally, everyone works together towards a common goal. In recent years in the UK there have been major changes in the management of the health service and there is an abundant literature on the subject of management. Concepts and terms such as 'core value' or 'mission statement', have become enshrined in a new management language.

However, such concepts may not adequately take into account the propensity for human relationships to subvert the smooth running of an organisation and hence to block the fulfilling of 'mission statements' and to compromise 'core values'. The function of management must, of course, address conflict between the human cogs of the machine, aiming to creatively utilise the energy that such conflicts generate or, alternatively, to devise systems for resolving or diffusing them. In the process, however, the relevant issues need not be oversimplified nor need the relationships involved become dehumanised.

Management, however, often deals with the problems of human interaction simply by construing them in public domain terms. Thus, for example, the significance of interstaff conflict is judged solely in terms of its effect on the smooth running of the organisation, not in terms of an interpersonal problem itself. The conflict may be accounted for in terms of mismatched or misaligned roles or functions, rather than in terms of the meanings the conflict may hold for the individuals concerned. In this way much of the emotional context of the conflict is bypassed or denied, and dealt with exclusively at a cognitive level. Time may be allowed for the ventilation of feelings but any remaining personal problems or problematic attitudes are left to the individuals to sort out for themselves, perhaps with an edict that these should not interfere with work. Often such management approaches are sufficient, but not always.

It was noticed that two non-clinical members of the clinic staff were at loggerheads in a way that generated sufficient bad feeling to affect everybody else working in the particular primary care practice. When the problem was addressed by the manager of the practice it became apparent that both parties felt the other should be undertaking some of the tasks they were in fact doing themselves. The problem was apparently solved by drawing up new and clearer job descriptions. However, within a month, the two were at loggerheads once more over another matter, unrelated to the first.

When problems are signalled by open and hostile conflict, as in the above example, they are easy for all to see. In such instances almost everyone recognises that the problem is really an interpersonal one but hopes, more than expects, that a practical (public domain) approach will solve it. In this way the more difficult task of sorting out why two people cannot get along together is avoided. As long as the overall functioning of the wider system is not seriously affected such a situation tends to be tolerated and the idea that the problematic relationship is but the symptom and not the disease is seldom entertained. Put another way, it is important to consider that the personal level of the interaction, as a potential source of problems, may require attention separate from, or in addition to, the more public domain aspects of the professional relationship. Problems, however, may be much more subtle and difficult to locate than in the above example and more damaging in their impact.

In another primary care clinic, it only gradually became apparent that important clinical screening data were not being collected and recorded. At a meeting of all staff, clinical and non-clinical, it had been agreed to collect the relevant information, apparently without any resistance. When the omission was reported at a subsequent clinical audit meeting everybody, once more, agreed to their alloted tasks but still the problem persisted. A rigorous investigation, as part of the auditing process, revealed that one of those involved was only intermittently collecting the required information. This was made clear to everyone and the culprit exposed. This resulted in various feelings of exasperation, contempt and shame.

This example of a persistent, i.e. significant and non-transitory, problem encountered in clinic management was finally revealed to reside more in the personal than in the public domain. Attempts to deal with such problems at the public level alone are therefore usually only partially successful. Fortunately, some of the modern literature on management grapples with these problems, for instance paying close attention to factors that facilitate or undermine motivation and commitment (Pringle *et al.*, 1991). This is recognised as especially important in the management of change.

Sometimes, as suggested above, conflict or incapacity to perform in some required aspect, is in fact a symptom of organisational structural problems within the clinic. Such problems can be most difficult and recalcitrant when they derive from the nature of medical work itself, i.e. from having to deal with painful frightening diseases, arousing feelings of disgust, fear, shame and grief, which mobilise powerful defensive mechanisms (Menzies-Lyth, 1970). Addressing them requires time and the involvement of staff with some psychological sophistication or training in psychodynamic and systemic processes. Nevertheless, incorporating a forum for the resolution of interstaff difficulties into the organisational structure of clinics, in order to deal with problems that arise out of working in the face of death and disease, can be most beneficial. Such forums can facilitate the discussions necessary to tease out which conflictual transactions result more as a symptom of an institutionalised malaise of the clinic or wider health care system than from interpersonal difficulties. Bearing this in mind, management perhaps should set up an organisational structure where difficult feelings and emotions inherent in the work, which evoke powerful defences, can be safely examined and potentially resolved. This is particularly important because the operation of the defences involved is likely to be unwitting and may manifest itself only in a disguised form in other problems that do surface.

Complicated transactions meeting

A suitable structure for the discussion and analysis of the interaction between complicated transactions and organisational functioning might take the form of regular meetings where such transactions, arising in the day-to-day work of the clinic, are examined using the methods described for the complicated clinical transaction, including utilising transaction and system windows.

At a primary care practice's clinical meeting one of the doctors provided a videotaped recording of a recent surgery. One of the consultations recorded was selected by a medical colleague, by stopping the tape at random, and the partners began to discuss it using the transaction window.

The patient, Mr Bingham, a fifty year old man, had attended on a number of occasions over several months. His presenting complaint had been of difficulty in passing urine, which the doctor diagnosed as due to an enlarged prostate gland. At the initial examination the doctor had become suspicious of prostatic cancer and the results of a blood test lent some support to this suspicion. He had consequently referred the patient for a specialist urological opinion.

It emerged, in the interim, that Mr Bingham was also depressed and anxious, voicing many domestic, financial and professional worries. An exploration of these concerns became the focus of subsequent consultations. In the consultation being watched, which the doctor concerned said was typical, Mr Bingham appeared hopeless and dejected and could see little prospect of his situation improving. As if in sympathy, the doctor's shoulders were drooped, his head lowered and his eyes averted. There were long periods of silence and both voices were muted and the interchange slow. The videotape was stopped.

Looking through the medical records, one of the partners commented that Mr Bingham had twice failed to attend his hospital out-patient urological appointment. This issue was not mentioned in the videotaped consultation nor, as Mr Bingham's doctor suddenly realised, in any of their recent meetings. He recalled having asked Mr Bingham about the matter after the first failure to attend but had not consciously registered the second missed appointment. The doctor was anxious about the delay so far entailed, as it might be of clinical significance, and shocked by the lapse of his attention it represented. As the partners pondered the personal level of the doctor–patient interaction, it was suggested that the doctor had become affected by Mr Bingham's depression and hopelessness, with the result that neither the management of a serious physical condition nor the diagnosis of an equally serious and potentially life-threatening depressive disorder had been clearly addressed.

Thinking about systemic influences, one of the partners asked if Mr Bingham's family knew of the seriousness of his prostatic problem. The doctor was unable to provide an answer to this but realised that here was at least an opportunity for breaking the stalemate and he resolved to ask Mr Bingham about this next time they met.

When they did next meet, it emerged that Mr Bingham had not told anyone else in the family about his referral to hospital, nor of the possible serious significance of his symptoms, although this had been clearly communicated by his doctor. He had sought to protect himself from the anxiety it aroused by denying it, either consciously or unconsciously. After this consultation Mr Bingham managed to discuss matters with his family and to keep his further hospital appointment. His wife accompanied him on his subsequent visit to his primary care doctor and, at least initially, also supervised his taking a course of anti-depressant medication. At operation, the prostate was removed and histology revealed no malignant changes. Mr Bingham's mood and personal functioning returned to normal over the next three months and his various worries gradually subsided.

The value of meetings such as the above is potentially twofold. First, clinical colleagues can share attitudes, feelings and information (with each other and other relevant personnel) and examine complicated clinical transactions in which they themselves are involved, both with a view to determining future actions and also looking for evidence of the impact of particular complicated clinical transactions on other systems in the clinic or the wider health care system of the practice or hospital. Second, other non-clinical transactions taking place within the clinical setting can be examined, not only with a view to resolving non-clinical personnel or management problems but also to search for evidence of their impact on the clinical transaction itself.

If such interlinked problems are to be tackled at anything more than a superficial level, a forum must be created that fosters and facilitates relationships of mutual trust and respect. Furthermore, the importance of such an endeavour must be acknowledged and accepted by all those involved. Beyond this, some knowledge and experience of the psycho-dynamics of the personal level of staff–patient and staff–staff interaction is necessary. This can be developed within the staff group but it may be beneficial to involve an independent facilitator with appropriate quali-fications, who can at regular intervals attend the clinic's complicated transactions meeting. Such an enterprise would be greatly facilitated if the doctors, in the course of their training, were primed for the task, for example by developing the skills involved in monitoring countertrans-ference reactions and identifying potentially adverse systemic influences, as discussed in earlier chapters. (Meetings to discuss problems posed by certain 'problem' patients represent a familiar development, as described in Chapter 1. Complicated transaction meetings would differ from these by virtue of the application of the conceptual framework and associated attributes that have been developed in this book.)

Conclusions

The health service as a system, together with all of its subsystems, is structured and functions, in part, to contain society's anxiety in respect to issues to do with intimacy, health, illness and death. The ways in which such anxieties are manifested and responded to varies according to the level within the hierarchy of systems that is under scrutiny. At the level of the clinical transaction between doctor and patient, these anxieties bear the personal trademark of doctor and patient (their personalities and habitual defensive strategies to deal with anxiety) as they perform their respective social roles. At higher levels in the hierarchy (managerial and governmental), the personal imprint may be less evident or distinctive and yet still subtly be present, since many of the relevant systems within the hierarchy are person-systems. As a result, even though seemingly public level activities, such as the strategic planning of the nation's health service, are being pursued, personal aspects of the professional personnel involved may emerge, often without their being recognised or acknowledged as such, which affect the process of discussion or negotiation and the securing of relevant goals for the service.

The same applies at the level of the clinic, albeit on a smaller scale and lower in the hierarchy. At the level of the individual clinic, the setting is superficially an impersonal entity with physical non-human structural elements. However, even these public domain aspects are not without a personal impact in terms of what is conveyed, both to patients and staff who use the clinic. The latter, of course, also comprises person-systems of two main types – one which involves patients and one which does not. The two systems, although conventionally conceived as being quite separate from one another, being person-systems and open (at least potentially so) to the influence of other such systems, may influence one another, sometimes adversely. The influence on the clinical transaction between doctor and patient (or between other clinical staff and patients) may be sufficiently adverse as to complicate it. Commonly this is via the direct or indirect expression of personal factors deriving from the doctor–patient interaction that cause complications, evidence for which arises in the personal domain itself or in the public domain or sometimes in both simultaneously.

In an analogous way, the staff–staff transaction (concerning clinical and non-clincal, professional matters) can be adversely affected by the eruption of personal aspects that impair the participants' capacities to perform satisfactorily their public level social roles as professionals. Thus staff–staff transactions may also be conceived as being straightforward or complicated. When the latter, they may act as adverse systemic influences potentially complicating one or more of the clinical transactions being undertaken. The whole clinic is thus an interacting mesh of systems that may affect one another and it has the potential to increase the overall level of complicated transactions within it.

Doctors, by virtue of being members of most of the overlapping and hierarchical subsystems of a clinic, are well placed to be influential in promoting or preventing complications within the system. It is perhaps appropriate, therefore, that they own responsibility for monitoring the clinic, from a systemic standpoint, and for setting in place any necessary structures (for example, complicated transactions meetings) that may be used in the service of recognising, analysing and resolving complicated transactions as they arise, which inevitably they will.

There is no single organisational structure that is best to deal with a particular clinic's complicated transactions; hence none is especially advocated here. The clinic system itself needs to negotiate a structure that works for itself. What is required, therefore, no matter what the structure might be, is a mechanism that can act to monitor, recognise and analyse complicated transactions into the component public and personal domains. These need to be separately understood so as to permit a fuller understanding of the interaction between the two domains. Only in this way can the interface between the clinical transaction and its human and systemic contexts be considered so as to minimise the influences that would otherwise serve to increase the pressures on clinical transactions to become complicated.

Although certain transactions within the clinic, for example those concerned with administrative matters, are influenced by public domain factors which are not directly clinical, it may nevertheless be beneficial for medical staff to be included in meetings established to consider them. Any causal links between potentially adverse systemic influences of the wider clinical setting and the clinical transaction itself may thus be more readily identified. In this way, the non-clinical and clinical systems within the clinic are kept in open communication with one another.

New structural forms may be required to achieve the above. Alternatively, the function may be subsumed under an existing structure, for example one of the clinic's existing meetings. Likewise, it may or may not be considered necessary to involve external, i.e. non-clinic, personnel versed in systemic thinking to provide some overall support or supervision.

9

Implications for training

Introduction

At pre-clinical, clinical and postgraduate levels, medical training could incorporate teaching on: the concept of straightforward and complicated clinical transactions; an understanding of the influence of personality and unconscious, as opposed to conscious, motivation of doctor and patient in their clinical interaction; the influence of past relationships with authority figures upon the attitudes and behaviour of doctor and patient as they transact; the influence of the psychological and social context (including the clinical setting itself) of doctor and patient on the clinical transaction; and the use of transaction and systems windows, as well as other interventions. This is because, particularly in primary care practice, it has long been acknowledged that diagnosis should be couched not only in physical but in psychological and social terms (Royal College of General Practitioners, 1972) and that the psychological component of the consultation is fundamental (Pendleton, 1983).

The work of Michael and Enid Balint (see Balint, 1957; Balint and Norrell, 1973), emphasising a deeper level of diagnosis, has influenced the practice of many doctors and, increasingly, doctors' attitudes to their patients form an important discriminator between 'good' and 'bad' doctors (Kilpatrick, 1993). It has also been recognised that doctors' interventions exert a psychological effect on patients that can influence the outcome of the clinical transactions not only in the short term but also in the long term (Freeling and Harris, 1984).

Even though, in the view of some (GMC, 1980; Samuel, 1990) the medical students' curriculum is already full, the teaching of additional topics concerning complicated clinical transactions could be integrated with students' existing training, which, for the most part, would require only a shift of emphasis and a demonstration of how such aspects fitted into the overarching conceptual model of the complicated clinical transaction. Likewise, for qualified doctors, who often have difficulty finding time for further training or study on account of long working hours, the implications of an understanding of complicated clinical transactions could readily harmonise with some of the existing theoretical and practical teaching that is provided. Possible ways in which teaching could be integrated at pre-clinical, clinical and postgraduate levels are described below.

Content of teaching

Pre-clinical stage

Pre-clinical courses for medical students already allocate time for the teaching of selected areas within the fields of psychology and sociology. However, such aspects are not necessarily appreciated to have a direct bearing on the clinical practice that follows during later training and beyond. Currently, there is the potential for the relevant information thus acquired to become compartmentalised and not to be readily accessible or to inform later clinical practice. In part this is because of the absence of an overarching conceptual model that brings together the relevant aspects, psychological and social, and integrates them with the thinking and practice that pertain to the actual clinical encounter. The concept of the straightforward or complicated clinical transaction, as defined and discussed in this book, represents a model that can fill the current gap and in so doing it emphasises and integrates specific aspects of psychology and sociology, making them more relevant and, perhaps, also more interesting. Thus, notions such as personality, transference–countertransference, sick role, medical model, and social network may be seen to bear a direct relevance to the doctor–patient relationship. Any additional theoretical and practical topics that would need to be acquired would not be simply extra baggage for the already encumbered student or doctor but represent vehicles for bringing together various existing strands of knowledge, attitudes and skills.

Clinical training

As at present, the clinical student would need to become proficient in obtaining, where relevant, a detailed psychosocial history. However, the aims of this could be made more clearly: to identify potentially conflicting goals, resulting from overlapping system membership; to identify prevailing attitudes and behaviours towards important other people in the patient's life, past and present (especially parents, partners and own children); and to identify adverse personality influences. All these aspects may serve to complicate a clinical transaction.

The social history must be elicited so as to determine whether, for example, the patient's work situation is producing demands on him or her that conflict with the smooth pursuit of the patient role. The pressure of financial difficulties, as another area, may be highly pertinent and require tactful and appropriate enquiry. The patient's living accommodation, in a way analogous to that of the doctor's clinical work environment, may affect his or her capacity to comply with specific requirements of treatment. Hence the doctor will need the requisite skills to efficiently obtain a snapshot of the patient in his or her usual social environment through relevant history-taking.

Taking a family history may enable the doctor to assess the quality of the patient's relationships with earlier authority figures, especially parents, since the pattern of such early relationships often endures and colours current relationships, including that with the doctor. Discovering a history of insecure or disorganised early attachments to parents can sensitise the doctor to the possibility of such a development within the clinical transaction that could be sufficient to complicate it. Pervading idiosyncratic family attitudes or culturally determined unusual attitudes to specific illness or to illness in general may be detected via appropriate questioning. Not only may such views be at odds with those of the doctor but they may also colour the patient's views of the doctor and hence affect the use such patients are able to make of doctors and the health system in general. Any clashes between 'lay' medical beliefs and those of the doctor can only be resolved once the differences have been openly acknowledged. Only then can the issues form part of the more routine public domain activity of the clinical transaction.

The quality of the patient's relationship with a current partner and with his or her own children may also provide pointers to factors that may complicate the clinical transaction with the doctor. The mechanism may be due to such adverse factors acting as direct stressors on the patient; producing conflict through divided loyalties resulting from overlapping system membership or representing a characteristic style of interaction that also becomes enacted with the doctor. Both of these routes may lead to a complicated clinical transaction.

Evidence of an abnormal personality may be obvious, as in the case of a patient with diagnosable personality disorder. Often, however, this will not be the case and questions aimed at revealing the patient's pre-morbid

Table 9.1. *Personality assessment headings*

Description of patient during interview
Enquiry for specific personality traits
    The effect of these traits upon personal relationships
    Illustration of personality traits in anecdotes from history
Social relationships
Activities and interests enjoyed
Predominant mood
Attitudes and values
Initiative and drive
Habits

personality and any relevant abnormalities will need to be asked. Patients, of course, may not always be reliable witnesses and collateral information from other informants, with the patient's permission, forms a useful additional source of information that can aid the doctor in making a diagnosis of personality disorder or not. Many patients, however, are able to provide valid information in response to appropriate questions. The latter need to address a variety of aspects (see Table 9.1 and Appendix II).

With practice all the above aspects of history-taking concerning personality assessment can be acquired and, while a detailed psychosocial enquiry will be beyond the compass of clinical students early on in the clinical stage of training, later the complexities of patients and their interpersonal and social contexts should be understandable.

Abnormalities in a patient's mental state may be obvious at interview or form part of the presenting complaint. Alternatively, they may emerge during history-taking in relation to another, perhaps somatic, complaint. Such abnormalities may also emerge during questioning regarding social and other interpersonal functioning as part of the psychosocial history-taking just described. When present, they may require the doctor's attention in their own right, whether or not they form part of a psychiatric disorder. As already discussed (in Chapter 6), in certain situations when the clinical transaction has become complicated, it is important to explore the patient's psychosocial situation and this may include a mental state examination, which in many cases can be brief. For the purpose of teaching clinical medical students, however, a thorough training in mental state examination is required (see Table 9.2) and this usually takes place during the formal psychiatric component of training. Only once a thorough understanding of mental state phenomena has been acquired,

Table 9.2. *Mental state headings*

Appearance and behaviour
Physical appearance (including posture and movement); consciousness and attention; dress; and behaviour in interview situation

Form of talk
Rate, quantity, continuity, coherence, pauses, use of words and syntax
(Recorded verbatim samples of speed can be helpful)

Mood
Subjective description of mood; objective assessment of mood

Thought content
Predominant thoughts and mood (morbid thoughts and suicidal ideas); disturbance of thought processes; obsessional ideas or compulsive acts; phobias; body image

Abnormal beliefs
Ideas of reference; misinterpretations; overvalued ideas; delusions

Abnormal perceptions
Pain; illusions; hallucinations; depersonalisation and derealisation

Cognitive function
Orientation; long-term memory; registration and short-term memory; immediate memory; attention and concentration; general information; current affairs; abstract thinking; intelligence

Patient's insight into illness and reaction to it

Doctor's reaction to patient

---

and the student is practiced at eliciting such aspects (especially those to do with suicidal ideation, psychotic phenomena, and cognitive impairment), are students in a position to take acceptable 'short-cuts', to know which are the essential or relevant areas on which to focus attention. Clearly a detailed mental state is neither appropriate nor desirable in the majority of cases of patients presenting with non-psychiatric complaints.

Postgraduate training

Having been educated within the hypothetical system of training described above, the emerging doctor will have been equipped to recognise a complicated clinical transaction and to understand how it can be differentiated from the straightforward clinical transaction and, also, to have acquired skills in the utilisation of transaction and systems windows. However, there may have been relatively little time to explore or obtain experience in ways in which complicated clinical transactions can be managed. In order to meet this training requirement the doctor's skills will need further refinement through specific attention to, and practice in, the supervised management of complicated clinical transactions. Obviously, for this to happen requires that the trainers themselves be suitably acquainted with, and experienced in, the model.

It is probably unrealistic to imagine that too much time and energy in the years immediately following qualification can be directed toward dealing with complicated clinical transactions as a topic for education. However, during postgraduate training there is no reason why such training should not appear in the curriculum. Doctors working in primary care settings in the UK already receive training that is highly developed in its teaching of doctor–patient communication and clinical interviewing skills. Thus, the incorporation of teaching about complicated clinical transactions, according to the model proposed here, would represent both a simple and logical development. In particular, the implied attitude required of doctors, in order more fully to take account of the personal level of the interaction and its supporting function in regard to the public level, is already advocated (GMC, 1987; Kilpatrick, 1993).

Experienced clinicians, previously relatively unaware of some of the ideas discussed in this book and of their synthesis in the form of the concept of the complicated clinical transaction, may also acquire such information at the postgraduate stage as part of their continuing professional development. Obtaining the relevant experience is possible in isolation but probably easier to assimilate through discussion with colleagues acquainted with the model. Therefore, informal or formal meetings to discuss the model and its application represent a possible teaching aid (see Chapter 8).

Teaching processes

Teaching about straightforward and complicated clinical transactions, the use of transaction and systems windows, and the management of complicated clinical transactions requires different processes at different stages of training. At the pre-clinical stage this will be largely didactic teaching of theory via a traditional lecture and seminar format and would require no change to existing teaching techniques. Obviously, videotaped clinical transactions could be used to exemplify the main points of the theory relevant at that stage, namely the recognition of the two types of clinical transaction and the use of the transaction window to elucidate the mechanism of the interplay between public and personal levels of the interaction between doctor and patient.

When students reach the clinical stage of training, methods would need to include actual doctor–patient interaction but the traditional teaching methods of assessing patients under the supervision of a trainer, as well as by observational learning from peers and seniors, would still be appropriate. However, time would be required in order to demonstrate the use of transaction and systems windows as aids to the monitoring and understanding of clinical transactions. Such teaching could occur either on an individual basis, between a single student and trainer, or via a small group of students supervised by a senior group leader. Role play techniques, the use of audiotape and videotape could all be utilised and it would be desirable to have teaching sessions devoted solely to the issues of complicated clinical transactions and their management.

The requirements for postgraduate level teaching represent an extension of those for clinical student training and, likewise, require separate attention being focussed on them. The precise method of teaching will depend upon the clinical setting in which the doctor works, whether there has been prior familiarity with the concepts and techniques, and upon the availability and co-operation of clinical colleagues. Certainly, with practice and experience, transaction and systems windows can be utilised by the single-handed practitioner in monitoring the clinical transactions. However, when the doctor is locked into a complicated clinical transaction with a patient, it can be useful to discuss the situation with a colleague or colleagues either on an as-required basis or as part of a regular monitoring of such transactions through the establishment of complicated clinical transaction meetings. The latter system confers certain advantages, specifically the possibility of prevention and early detection of complicated transactions. However, such a regular meeting may not be a feasible option for all doctors interested in applying the relevant concepts. In discussing the personal aspects of the doctor that may contribute to the development of complicated clinical transactions, a close and confiding working liaison with colleagues who are used to discussing complicated clinical transactions and their own personal contributions to them, can be beneficial (see below).

During training in primary care, it is common for trainer and trainee to sit in and observe each other's clinical practice.

In one such clinic, in which the trainer was observing, they took time after the clinic had finished to discuss one of the consultations. A young mother had brought her toddler, who was miserable because of an earache associated with an acute upper respiratory tract infection. All went well initially and the trainee carefully examined the child. Finding no signs of middle ear or chest infection he suggested to the mother that no treatment other than simple analgesia was required, since the infection, caused by a virus, would resolve on its own. The mother appeared obviously unhappy with this advice and asked if the child should have an antibiotic as well. The trainee began to show signs of feeling uncomfortable, but reiterated the advice, expanding the explanation of his understanding of the illness and its treatment. Reluctantly the child's mother accepted this and asked for a prescription for paracetamol syrup. Looking decidedly uncomfortable the trainee said that a suitable preparation could be bought over the counter without a prescription. Mother and child left, with both the mother and the trainee looking unhappy with the outcome of the transaction.

Such a transaction is common enough in primary care settings and the trainer took the opportunity, using transaction and system windows, to analyse it with the trainee in some detail. They constructed windows together, filling in boxes and indicating interactive processes with arrows as they went along (Figure 9.1).

Assessment

The assessment of clinical skills, whether of students or qualified doctors, is potentially problematic. However, the theoretical aspects of complicated clinical transactions and the related techniques and interventions could all be tested via traditional methods, whether by multiple choice question, short answer question, essay or viva voce. The practical application of such concepts may be harder to test partly because they represent specific attitudes and aspects of the doctor's style. In part, difficulty follows from the fact that a complicated clinical transaction is the result of a unique combination and interplay of patient and clinician factors. Hence the candidate cannot be presented with a complicated clinical transaction unless this has been artificially arranged. The artificiality introduced could clearly impair the validity of the assessment process. However, it might be possible to envisage stooge patients, professional actors, performing in such a way as to test the relevant skills of candidates. Alternatively, the use of appropriately selected video-taped interactions between doctors and patients (or stooge patients) could be shown to candidates, as brief clinical vignettes. Candidates could then discuss with examiners how to construe, in terms of the complicated clinical transaction model, the

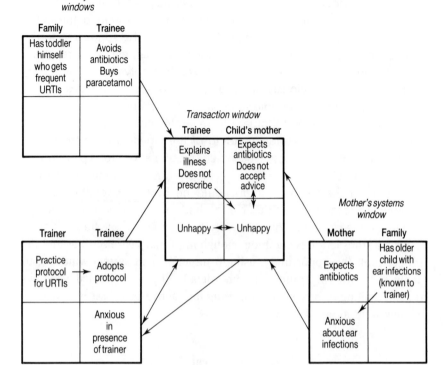

Figure 9.1. Transaction and systems windows indicating the interaction between trainer, trainee and child's mother. URTI, upper respiratory tract infection.

observed clinical interaction with specific focus on the identification of public and personal domains and their potential interplay. Candidates could also discuss where they might logically intervene were they faced with such a complicated clinical transaction in terms of the information yielded by the application of the transaction and systems windows. Thus, management issues relating to complicated transactions could also be appropriately discussed and assessed.

Conclusions

In learning about complicated clinical transactions, through the teaching process described above, medical students and doctors would necessarily become more aware of their contributions to the clinical transaction and, in particular, how their own personal aspects might serve to complicate it. The doctor's impact on the clinical transaction is at one and the same time as a representative of a societal system, via performing the social role of doctor, and as an individual person. There is thus the potential for a clash of interests or goals resulting from the interplay between the two levels of interaction. Many of the processes that govern interactions between people, including that between doctor and patient, are unconscious. Paradoxically, beyond a certain point (different for different individuals) the greater the disparity between the goals of the two domains, public and personal, the greater the likelihood that the difference will be defended against and not directly experienced (see Psychological defence mechanisms, Chapter 3, p. 42). Even when personal factors, such as a degree of physical attraction between doctor and patient, come into awareness their existence or importance is often minimised. Many factors thus contribute to keeping the personal domain silent and invisible and indeed this may be entirely appropriate in the majority of clinical transactions. However, once the transaction has become complicated, such aspects are ignored at the doctor's peril, since they may importantly contribute to the continuing of the complication of the transaction, the more so the longer they remain unrecognised or unacknowledged. For some doctors, taking into account such aspects requires a shift in basic attitude towards their work environment, working practice, their patients and how they view themselves, hence the need for a relevant and coherent conceptual model.

Doctors work in many different settings, both clinical and non-clinical, and the demands of their posts will tax them differently in terms of their performance in the public and personal domains. In many instances, the work with patients is but one facet and there are many other transactions with clinical and non-clinical colleagues, with carers of patients and with patients' families. In the UK collaborative working with management is also, increasingly, a feature of working as a doctor in the health system. How the clinical setting is structured and organised will affect the clinical transaction and this influence needs to be appreciated. Optimally, deciding on how best to organise the work setting rests upon a conceptual model, such as that described in this book.

It is impossible to predict how health care services will develop in the future. However, it would seem that a knowledge of the interaction of their component subsystems, both clinical and non-clinical, is important if future developments are to be governed by more than financial or economic factors. Conflicting goals, at different hierarchical levels within the overall healthcare system, can complicate the management of the individual patient. The importance of effective lines of communication are therefore crucial if goals of different hierarchical levels are to be, none the less, compatible. Equally important, however, is the maintenance of boundaries between hierarchical levels so that any conflict specific to a particular level is solved there and does not 'leak' to other levels within the organisation. The assimilation of the ideas presented in this book may provide doctors, and other staff, with a model that they can apply not only to the understanding of clinical transactions with patients but also to the organisations in which they work.

Appendix I

Clinical phenomena related to 'problem patients'

Somatisation

Somatisation is a tendency to express and communicate somatic distress and symptoms unaccounted for by pathological findings, to attribute them to physical illness and to seek medical help for them. Consequently, somatising patients are those who frequently complain of physical symptoms that either lack demonstrable organic bases or are judged to be grossly in excess of what one would expect on the grounds of objective medical findings (Lipowski, 1988). Such patients are commonly encountered in both primary and secondary care settings.

Somatisation, of course, does not imply that the patient does not have a concurrent physical or mental illness. On the contrary, in some cases it can actually coexist with, mask or be facilitated by such an illness (McFarland *et al.*, 1985). Overall, it is the pattern of predominantly somatic rather than cognitive response to stress and related emotional arousal that is the common feature of somatising patients. Such highly somatic responders display a wide diversity of physical symptoms and psychological characteristics and have been shown to make greater use of health care services than do low somatic responders (Frost *et al.* 1986). Somatising patients pose obvious problems for the doctors seeking to treat them, who might wish to avoid colluding in the management of a physical illness they regard as non-existent and yet they may be unable to convince their patients of the accuracy of this assessment.

Somatisation does not encompass all physical symptoms unaccounted for by demonstrable physical illness. Nor should somatisation be considered abnormal or a medical or psychiatric problem per se since the tendency to experience and communicate distress in a somatic rather than a psychosocial mode is widespread in Western and other societies (Kirmayer, 1984). It becomes a problem, however, when individuals who are so disposed attribute their somatic symptoms to physical illness and consequently seek medical diagnosis and treatment, especially so when they present persistently despite doctors' reassurances that physical illness cannot account for their symptoms.

Somatisation may occur at any age and is not excessively common in the elderly (Lipowski, 1988). It is not clear whether either sex predominates (Slavney and Teitelbaum, 1985). It is a common problem in health care as evidenced by clinical and epidemiological studies. In a large North American study (Wallen *et al.*, 1987), involving 327 hospitals and over 260 000 patients, 5.2 per cent were placed in the diagnostic category of 'symptoms and ill-defined

155

conditions', most of whom would fall into the category of being somatisers. In another large study of primary care practice, a survey looked at 90 000 visits to doctors and found that, of 72 per cent of the patients who received psychiatric diagnoses, each had one or more physical symptoms as the chief complaint (Schurman *et al.*, 1985). Other studies have found that approximately 30 per cent of primary care patients using health care services in a given year have diagnosable psychiatric disorders, most often depressive or anxiety disorders, and over half of them present with somatic rather than psychological symptoms (Parker *et al.*, 1984; Bridges and Goldberg, 1985; Kessler *et al.* 1985). One study, however, found that many of such patients did not attribute their somatic symptoms to physical illness when interviewed by psychiatrists, even though they had implied such attributions in their contacts with the primary physicians (Bridges and Goldberg, 1985). Such patients as these have been referred to as 'facultative' rather than 'true' somatisers. For them the physical complaint is utilised as an opening gambit in the context of consulting a doctor. True somatisers, by contrast, may well reject any suggestion that their physical symptomatology is a response to psychosocial stress.

Somatisation and psychiatric diagnosis

Somatisation does not represent a specific diagnostic category nor does it imply that a diagnosable psychiatric disorder must be present. It may, for example, occur as a transient stress response, one that hardly warrants a psychiatric diagnostic label (Lipowski, 1988). However, somatisation may be associated with a wide range of psychiatric disorders. Somatisation may be: a primary problem (as in so-called somatoform disorders); associated with a readily diagnosable non-somatoform psychiatric disorder, for example major depression; a 'masked disorder', as in the case of so-called masked depression; or a personality trait (Escobar *et al.*, 1987). The range of possibilities has obvious relevance to the management of patients who present as somatisers.

All abnormal emotional states involve physiological concomitants, any or all of which the person may perceive as symptoms and selectively focus on. It is such selective focussing that characterises the somatiser (Lipowski, 1988). On the other hand, an emotionally distressed person may selectively present physical complaints to a doctor on the assumption that this is the best approach to secure relief for the psychological distress. If properly and comprehensively interviewed, however, some such patients may speak freely of their psychosocial problems and, as indicated above, strictly speaking they should not be viewed as somatisers.

A positive association between somatisation and depressive disorders has been documented by clinical and epidemiological studies (Wilson *et al.*, 1982; Parker *et al.*, 1984; Bridges and Goldberg, 1985; Blacker and Clare, 1987). Depression is claimed to be one of the most common causes of somatisation (Katon *et al.*, 1982) and approximately three quarters of the patients who seek medical care for depressive illness do so in primary care settings (Prestidge and Lake, 1987). The majority of them complain of somatic rather than psychological distress and symptoms (Parker *et al.*, 1984; Bridges and Goldberg, 1985).

Somatisation is also associated with anxiety disorders. Patients suffering from panic disorder tend to consult non-psychiatric physicians and are likely to be misdiagnosed by them (Katon, 1984). They commonly present with various somatic complaints, such as chest pain, palpitations, dyspepsia, headache, dizziness, fainting and dyspnoea. Several factors have been proposed to account for somatisation in anxiety disorders. Enhanced awareness of and selective attention to bodily sensations and danger-related information generally (Macleod *et al.*, 1986), increased sympathetic nervous system arousal and patients' negative bias in appraising their health (Noyes *et al.*, 1986) have all been invoked as factors facilitating somatisation in anxious patients. As in the case of depression, the diagnosis of an anxiety disorder in a somatiser who denies emotional distress still rests on formal diagnostic criteria, but distinguishing it from somatisation disorder (APA, 1987) may be particularly difficult (Katon, 1984).

Psychosis of various types may feature somatic or hypochondriacal delusions of having a physical disease or of a body change, malfunction, or deformity. Some of these delusions may be focussed on a single theme, for example, as in parasitosis. A psychotic patient may, however, seek medical help for somatic symptoms, such as pain or weakness, lacking organic explanation but not elaborated in a delusional manner. Many schizophrenic patients are reported to do so (Varsamis and Adamson, 1976).

Denial of physical illness

As noted in Chapter 1, another category of patients who are difficult to manage is those who display pathological denial in relation to their physical illness (Groves, 1978). There is a literature on this topic that is focussed on differing aspects: the classification of denial (Vaillant, 1971), its psychological function (Douglas and Druss, 1987), and its quantification (Hackett and Cassem, 1974). The term has been variously applied and misused (Shelp and Perl, 1985) and this, in part, stems from the absence of a standard definition of denial itself (Cousins, 1982).

Confusion over the definition has led to a wide range of reported frequency in samples of medically ill patients (Strauss *et al.*, 1990). Denial may at times refer to the illness itself and at other times to its implications, including death (Weisman, 1972). Attempts to bring clarity to the situation include assessment of, for example, the disavowal of reality and the absence of anxiety (Havik and Maeleund, 1986).

There is no consensus about whether the terms 'healthy' and 'pathological' denial refer to the extent to which reality is disavowed, the degree to which an expected affect is absent or to outcome (Strauss *et al.*, 1990). Denial, for example, in cardiac patients (Hackett *et al.*, 1968) and cancer patients (Greer *et al.*, 1979) may be adaptive. However, there is a suggestion that it is other aspects of the patients, for example their overall approach to life, that is the key determinant of outcome (Beisser, 1979; Kobasa, 1982; Druss and Douglas, 1988).

It is not uncommon for patients to be referred to psychiatrists because they refuse to accept treatment for a physical condition (Strauss *et al.*, 1990). In such cases it is important to distinguish denial from other clinical scenarios in which treatment may be refused: patients who are unable to comply with treatment or lifestyle changes because of the implication that compulsive or additive behaviour (drugs, alcohol or smoking) has to be overcome; patients who habitually demonstrate poor judgment and/or impulsivity as part of their personalities; patients with health care belief systems of a subculture that may be in disagreement with proposed medical treatment.

The term 'denial' is in common usage among medical staff and it would seem that, in primary health care, as well as in hospital practice settings, the category of patients who would fall within the 'denial of a physical illness', as defined above (Strauss *et al.*, 1990), forms an important subgroup of those whom doctors find difficult to manage. It would appear that at least some doctors are aware of the pitfalls of using the term 'denial', particularly in using it in an undefined manner. Baseline management of such patients would dictate a thorough physical and psychosocial evaluation and full discussion of diagnosis, treatment and prognosis.

Hysteria

Like the term 'denial', 'hysteria' has been used in many different senses, for example synonymously with somatisation (Lipowski, 1988). The following have been identified (Kendell, 1972): conversion hysteria, the hysterical personality, Briquet's syndrome, mass hysteria, anxiety hysteria and 'an unsatisfactory doctor/patient relationship'. Consequently, there have been many critics of the term 'hysteria' and of its use by doctors (Slater, 1965; Mace, 1992). 'Dissociative states' has been the preferred term to refer to fugues, amnesias, tremors, pareses, anaesthesias, etc. (WHO, 1978). However, dissociative symptoms should not be taken as being the same as hysteria, since they may be seen in association with functional and organic illness or syndromes, including those causing more or less direct changes to cerebral physiology. Too often the diagnosis of hysteria is a way of avoiding a confrontation with the doctors' ignorance and 'the diagnosis of "hysteria" applies to a disorder of the doctor–patient relationship' (Slater, 1965). A recent historical review and critique of hysterical conversion confirms the inconsistent use of this term but argues for its continued presence in diagnostic classifications (Mace, 1992).

Patients may present dissociative or conversion 'symptoms' to doctors in primary care settings in the absence of demonstrable organic pathology and prove to be difficult to manage. With regard to the use of the term 'hysteria', caution should be exercised. Doctors should entertain the possibility of their own ignorance of patients and their conditions and also an awareness of themselves in relation to their patients.

Hypochondriasis

Hypochondriasis is a term used variously, for example to refer to a personality trait, a symptom (Kenyon, 1964), or an independent disease (Gillespie, 1929; APA, 1987). Confusingly, it has been used, at times, interchangeably with hysteria and somatisation (Lipowski, 1988). Its status as a disease entity on its own remains the subject of debate and there have been various conceptualisations of the phenomenon; psychodynamic, interpersonal, behavioural and cognitive (Barsky and Wyshak, 1990). A cognitive view suggests that the hypochondriac 'amplifies' a wide range of sensations: normal physiological factors, the benign symptoms of trivial and self-induced ailments, the somatic concordants of emotional disorder, as well as the symptoms of significant disease.

Like hysteria, hypochondriasis carries with it pejorative overtones. In spite of this it is likely that many patients whom doctors find difficult to manage will continue to acquire the label hypochondriac or hypochondriacal. A recent controlled study of psychological treatment in hypochondriasis recommended the retention of the category of hypochondriasis (Barsky *et al.*, 1992). Hypochondriacs in this study, from a general medical clinic, compared to non-hypochondriacs in the same setting showed significantly increased psychiatric morbidity, including a threefold increase in cases of personality disorder in the hypochondriacs.

Alexithymia

Alexithymia (from Greek *a*, without; *lexis*, word; *thumos*, heart or affectivity) means having no words for feelings (Nemiah and Sifneos, 1970). The concept refers to a series of phenomena that includes not only difficulties patients may have in attempting to describe their emotional states but also an incapacity to distinguish one emotion from another, for example anger from depression. The apparent disavowal of affectivity is not limited to 'painful' emotions. Thus, there is also an inability to experience satisfaction and pleasure.

In its effect, an impediment such as alexithymia will impact upon patients' relationships especially with those in intimate contact. Not only are such patients unable to capture and become aware of their own emotional experience but they have equal difficulty in understanding other people's emotional states and wishes. They may thus induce in others interpersonal difficulties, the precise nature of which will depend upon characteristics, including the degree of alexithymia, of both parties. In the context of the doctor–patient interaction, somatic symptoms may be presented, as if substituting for an emotional complaint, without the patient's awareness of the fact and in the absence of actual physical pathology.

Munchausen's syndrome

Munchausen's syndrome (Asher, 1951) is a curious condition in which patients repeatedly seek medical help or hospital treatment for consciously or unconsciously feigned symptoms. The eponym Munchausen was chosen because of the similarities between the wandering and fabrications of such patients and the fantastic adventures and anecdotes attributed to Baron Munchausen (1720–1797). Presentation is often dramatic, with symptoms and history suggestive of an acute organic emergency, leading to concentrated medical care, admission and even surgery. Investigation and treatment serve only to reinforce the likelihood of recurring episodes. On the other hand, turning the patient away may serve the doctor's needs rather than those of the patient. The professional challenge remains to develop an appropriate medical response that seeks to identify and isolate the underlying problems and to help the patient cope with them. The full-blown syndrome is not commonly encountered in primary care settings but minor forms or variations are probably more common than is realised, involving as they may elements of somatisation, hysteria and hypochondriasis. Management of patients of this kind obviously benefits from careful collaboration between primary care physicians and secondary care specialists who are involved with a given patient.

In certain instances (Munchausen's syndrome by proxy) other people may be used by the patient in place of the presentation of symptoms as, for example, the case of a mother fabricating a complaint on behalf of her child (Meadow, 1977). Almost any clinical picture can be simulated but common presentations are epileptic seizures and infant apnoea. Psychiatric as well as physical symptoms or signs can be involved. An adult in a care-giving role, usually the parent of the child (and most commonly the mother), either fabricates a history or induces symptoms or signs, for example, by suffocation as a means of producing seizures or apnoea. Laboratory samples may be tampered with to mislead clinicians via abnormal investigative findings and children may be poisoned. The child is presented for medical care with the parent claiming no knowledge of the cause. The 'illnesses' are often prolonged and treatment ineffective. The mothers involved may have unusually close relationships with hospital staff and may have incomplete nurse training or other medical contacts. They appear to have few social outlets and uninvolved or emotionally distant partners. Some of the mothers may have features of Munchausen's syndrome, while others appear depressed or have a personality disorder (Fisher *et al.* 1993).

Malingering

The term 'malingerer' is usually reserved for patients who invite their doctors' scorn and disapprobation by wilfully fabricating illness to gain status or financial reward. The conscious abuse of the doctor–patient relationships marks malingering as different from hysteria or Munchausen's syndrome and yet it might be conceived as lying along a continuum that includes these as well as genuine complaints of illness. Whereas in hysteria the patient is entirely unconscious in formulating a complaint or symptom, in Munchausen's syndrome, motivation is less clearly unconscious and, indeed, has a conscious component. In the case of the malingerer, however, the patient is entirely conscious of the deceit that is perpetrated, even though the reasons for the deceit may not be clear.

Appendix II
Personality disorder

Definition

According to the International Classification of Diseases (WHO, 1992), personality disorder refers to conditions which comprise:

deeply ingrained and enduring behaviour patterns, manifesting themselves as inflexible responses to a broad range of personal and social situations. They represent either extreme or significant deviations from the way the average individual in a given culture perceives, thinks, feels and particularly relates to others. Such behaviour patterns tend to be stable and to encompass multiple domains of behaviour and psychological functioning. They are frequently, but not always, associated with various degrees of subjective distress and problems in social functioning and performance.

The other major classification scheme – *Diagnostic and statistical manual of mental disorders* (APA, 1987) – utilises very similar criteria. Thus, personality disorder is defined as:

behaviours or traits that are characteristic of the person's recent (past year) and long-term functioning (generally since adolescence or early adulthood). The constellation of behaviours or traits causes either significant impairment in social or occupational functioning or subjective distress. Behaviours or traits limited to episodes of illness are not considered in making a diagnosis of Personality Disorder.

Personality disorder subtypes

Subclassification is currently limited to the description of a series of types and subtypes that are not mutually exclusive and that overlap in some of their characteristics. In making a diagnosis of personality disorder, the clinician should consider all aspects of personal functioning, although the diagnostic formulation will refer only to those dimensions or traits for which suggested thresholds for severity are reached. The assessment should be based, ideally, on as many sources of information as possible. Although it is sometimes possible to evaluate a personality condition in a single interview with the patient, it is often necessary to have more than one interview and to collect history data from other informants. Subcategorisation of personality disorders is unreliable, especially where the condition is severe (Coid, 1990, 1992; Grove and Tellegen, 1991). Such severe cases (perhaps representing 2 per cent of the total population but representing a much heavier relative clinical demand on health services) obviously represent a small minority of patients seen, whether in primary or secondary care settings.

161

Personality disorder tends to appear in late childhood or adolescence and continues to be manifest into adulthood. It is therefore unlikely that the diagnosis of personality disorder will be appropriate before the age of sixteen or seventeen years. Such information needs to inform the clinician's history-taking and mental state examination. Evidence is required to demonstrate: markedly disharmonious attitudes and behaviour, involving several areas of functioning, for example impulse control and style of relating to others; an enduring pattern of abnormal behaviour not limited to episodes of illness; an abnormal behaviour pattern that is pervasive and clearly maladaptive to a broad range of personal and social situations; attitudes and behaviour that lead to considerable personal distress, which, however, may be apparent only later in the course of the disorder; an association with significant problems in occupational and social performance.

Table AII.1 displays a comparison of the ICD 10 and DSM-III-R classifications and provides brief descriptions that make clear some of the important subtypes of personality disorder (Tyrer, 1991).

Reported prevalence rates for personality disorder vary, but there is accumulating evidence for a prevalence of approximately 10 per cent of the total population (Reich *et al.*, 1989; Zimmerman and Coryell, 1989). Other research (Tyrer, 1988) has identified a gradient within the referral system to psychiatrists with increasing prevalence from 10 per cent of the general population increasing through general practice attenders (approximately 20 per cent) to psychiatric out-patient attenders (approximately 30 per cent) and to psychiatric in-patients (approximately 40 per cent). Corresponding data for prevalence of personality disorder in other medical conditions are lacking, although it is known that the addictions (to illicit drugs, prescribed drugs, alcohol and tobacco) are all positively associated with personality disorder. Likewise, disorders of eating (anorexia nervosa, bulimia nervosa, and obesity) are all over-represented in personality disordered individuals (Levin and Hyler, 1986; Pope *et al.*, 1987; Cooper *et al.*, 1988; Gartner *et al.*, 1989). The sexual behaviour of personality disordered individuals is also abnormal, spanning the major perversions and also including sexual victimisation, for example rape and child sexual abuse (Russell, 1983).

Personality disorder, as a primary diagnosis, represents 8.4 per cent of first psychiatric in-patient admissions in the UK and 7.2 per cent of all admissions to mental hospitals (Health and Personal Social Service statistics). Since secondary diagnoses are seldom reliably coded, the above figure represents an under-estimate of the true rates of personality disorder in such populations. A recently cited study of psychiatric in-patients (Casey, 1988) found that the rate of personality disorder increased from 15 to 50 per cent once *all* patients were screened for a personality disorder diagnosis.

The co-existence of personality disorder with other psychiatric illness (symptom disorder) diagnoses, for example, schizophrenia or manic-depressive psychosis, is not solely of academic interest. It is associated with poorer treatment response and longer, and hence more costly, treatment (Tyrer, 1988). The effect of personality disorder on the treatment of medical conditions is not known. Compliance with treatment is likely to be impaired, as is taking up of medical advice, the end result being more costly treatment.

There is no single cause of personality disorder. There are substantial associations between later personality disorder and earlier childhood influences such as: poor supervision, parental uninvolvement, parental criminality and aggressiveness, composite family handicap and deviant peers (Loeber, 1990;

Table AII.1. *Comparison of current classification of personality disorder*

ICD 10		DSM-III-R	
Code	Description	Code	Description
F60.0	*Paranoid* – excessive sensitivity, suspiciousness, preoccupation with conspiratorial explanation of events, with a persistent tendency to self-reference	301.00	*Paranoid* – interpretation of people's actions as deliberately demeaning or threatening
F60.1	*Schizoid* – emotional coldness. detachment, lack of interest in other people, eccentricity and introspective fantasy.	301.20	*Schizoid* – indifference to relationships and restricted range of emotional experience and expression
	No equivalent	302.22	*Schizotypal* – deficit in inter-personal relatedness with peculiarities of ideation, appearance and behaviour
F60.5	*Anankastic* – indecisiveness, doubt, excessive caution, pedantry, rigidity and need to plan in immaculate detail	301.40	*Obsessive–compulsive* – pervasive perfectionism and inflexibility
F60.4	*Histrionic* – self-dramatisation, shallow mood, egocentricity and craving for excitement with persistent manipulative behaviour	301.50	*Histrionic* – excessive emotionally and attention seeking
F60.7	*Dependent* – failure to take responsibility for actions, with subordination of personal needs to those of others, excessive dependence with need for constant reassurance and feelings of helplessness when a close relationship ends	301.60	*Dependent* – persistent dependent and submissive behaviour
F60.2	*Dyssocial* – callous unconcern for others, with irresponsibility, irritability and aggression, and incapacity to maintain enduring relationships	301.70	*Antisocial* – evidence of repeated conduct disorder before the age of 15 years
	No equivalent	301.81	*Narcissistic* – pervasive grandi-osity, lack of empathy, and hypersensitivity to the evaluation of others
F60.6	*Anxious* – persistent tension, self-consciousness, exaggeration of risks and dangers, hyper-sensitivity to rejection, and restricted lifestyle because of insecurity	301.82	*Avoidant* – pervasive social discomfort, fear or negative evaluation and timidity
F60.30	*Impulsive* – inability to control anger, to plan ahead, or to think before acts, with unpredictable mood and quarrelsome behaviour	301.83	*Borderline* – pervasive of mood, and self-image
F30.31	*Borderline* – unclear self-image, involvement in intense and unstable relationships	301.84	*Passive–aggressive* – pervasive passive resistance to demands for adequate social and occupational performance

Source: Tyrer, 1991.

Paris and Frank, 1989). There is also a positive association between personality disorder and previous child sexual abuse (Herman *et al.*, 1989) and alcohol and drug misuse by parents (Lewis and Bucholz, 1991). Aetiological agents exert their effect particularly via disturbed relationships with close family members during the formative years of the personality, mainly through long-term repeated influences rather than a single traumatic event. In this way, personality disordered parents often beget personality disordered offspring. Although difficult to quantify, the genetic contribution to this familial transmission of psychopathology is likely to be small (Widom, 1991)

Personality disorder as a determinant of health care-seeking behaviour

Many patients suffering from moderate to severe personality disorder have little tolerance of anxiety or other psychic (or physical) pain. They tend to present for help during a crisis, sometimes dramatically. The distortion of the personality, being the result of influences acting in childhood and adolescence, is such as to impair any capacity to trust authority figures including doctors and nurses (Gerstley *et al.*, 1989). This mistrust is rooted in a profoundly low self-esteem. One result is that harm, misfortune or illness is experienced as being deserved. Another outcome is that any real help provided is experienced as not merited. Hence compliance with treatment is poor. The result is episodes of incomplete treatment, hence poorer outcome (Perry *et al.*, 1987).

Personality disordered patients attempt to find other ways of dealing with anxiety or of bolstering poor self-esteem that centre on various maladaptive strategies – all of which may be also damaging (directly or indirectly) to others who come into relation to them (Perry and Klerman, 1980). Such strategies include short-term anxiety reduction by illicit or prescribed (e.g. benzodiazepine) drug misuse, alcohol dependence, eating disorders (anorexia nervosa, bulimia nervosa, obesity), tobacco smoking, sexual disinhibition (including prostitution and promiscuity) or physical aggression directed at the self or others. This can result in psychological damage or abuse of others and there may be associated physical abuse (both deliberate and via neglect) and an increased risk of human immunodeficiency virus/acquired immune deficiency syndrome (HIV/AIDS), on account of the sexual disinhibition and drug misuse.

Not surprisingly, personality disordered patients are difficult to engage in treatment. Their presentation to professionals is often by a self-damaging act (overdose, wrist-slashing, burning) or else via an act of delinquency (theft, violence) rather than by the presentation of a symptom such as depression or anxiety. To an extent, the traditional medical model demands a 'symptom' as a *sine qua non* for treatment. Many doctors therefore feel disempowered, professionally, by personality disordered patients who do not produce such an 'entry ticket'. Failure of the clinical encounter can lead to the maintenance of patients' mistrust of authority figures, on the one hand, and therapeutic nihilism from clinicians, on the other (Lewis and Appleby, 1988).

The first therapeutic challenge, therefore, is to facilitate the personality disordered individual in becoming a patient, i.e. a person who is capable of verbalising a complaint or symptom rather than expressing painful feelings via actions. 'Actions' do indeed speak louder than words but clinicians need to be able to delve below the level of actions (and indeed of symptoms) in order to address the underlying negative attitudes, which are at the root of the disorder of personality and which fuel the self-damaging and other maladaptive behaviours.

References

Abed, R. T. and Neira-Muñoz, E. (1990) A survey of general practitioners' opinions and attitudes to drug addicts and addiction. *British Journal of Addiction*, **85**, 131–6.

Abercrombie, W., Hill, S. and Turner, B. S. (1984) *The Penguin dictionary of sociology*. London: Penguin Books Ltd.

Adelman, S. (1983) Pills as transitional objects: a dynamic understanding of the use of medication in psychotherapy. *Psychiatry*, **48**, 246–53.

Agazarian, Y. and Peters, R. (1981) *The visible and invisible group*. London, New York: Routledge and Kegan Paul.

Ainsworth, M. D. S., Blehar, M. C., Waters, E. and Wall, S. (1978) *Patterns of attachment: a psychological study of the strange situation*. Hillsdale, NJ: Erlbaum.

APA (American Psychiatric Association) (1987) *Diagnostic and statistical manual of mental disorders*, 3rd edn rev. Washington, DC: APA.

Arber, S. and Sawyer, L. (1982) Do appointment systems work? *British Medical Journal*, **284**, 478–80.

Arber, S. and Sawyer, L. (1985) The role of the receptionist in general practice – a dragon at the desk. *Social Science and Medicine*, **20A**, 911–21.

Armstrong, D. (1986) Illness behaviour revisited. In *Proceedings of the 15th European Conference on Psychosomatic Research*, eds J. H. Lacey and D. A. Sturgeon, pp. 115–19. London: John Libbey & Co. Ltd.

Asher, R. (1951) Munchausen's syndrome. *Lancet*, **i**, 339–40.

Balint, E. and Norell, J. S. (1973) *Six minutes for the patient; interactions in general practice consultation*. London: Tavistock.

Balint, M. (1957) *The doctor, his patient, and the illness*. New York: International Universities Press.

Barsky, A. J. and Wyshak, G. (1990) Hypochondriasis and somatosensory amplification. *British Journal of Psychiatry*, **157**, 404–9.

Barsky, A. J., Wyshak, G. and Klerman, G. L. (1992) Psychiatric comorbidity in DSM-III-R hypochondriasis. *Archives of General Psychiatry*, **49**, 101–7.

Beisser (1979) Denial and affirmation in illness and health. *American Journal of Psychiatry*, **136**, 1026–30.

Blacker, C. V. R. and Clare, A. W. (1987) Depressive disorder in primary care. *British Journal of Psychiatry*, **150**, 737–51.

Blaxter, M. (1983) The cause of disease: women talking. *Social Science and Medicine*, **17**, 59–69.

Bowlby, J. (1958) The nature of the child's ties to his mother. *International Journal of Psychoanalysis*, **39**, 350–73.

Bridges, R. N. and Goldberg, D. P. (1985) Somatic presentation of DSM-III psychiatric disorders in primary care. *Journal of Psychosomatic Research*, **29**, 563–9.

Brier, J. and Zaidi, L. Y. (1989) Sexual abuse histories and sequelae in female psychiatric emergency room patients. *American Journal of Psychiatry*, **146**, 1602–6.

Bucks, R. S., Williams, A., Whitfield, J. and Routh, D. A. (1990) Towards a typology of general practitioners' attitudes to general medicine. *Social Science and Medicine*, **30**, 537–47.

Byrne, P. and Long, B. E. L. (1976) *Doctors talking to patients*. London: HMSO.

Calnan, M. (1988) Images of general practice: the perceptions of the doctor. *Social Science and Medicine*, **27**(6), 579–86.

Casey, P. (1988) In: *Personality disorders: diagnosis, management and cause*. ed. P. Tyrer, pp. 74–81. London: Wright.

Chesser, E. S. (1975) Psychosocial reactions to investigation and treatment of organic disease. *Medicine*, **10**(1), 447–52.

Coid, J. W. (1990) Psychopathic disorders. *Current Opinion in Psychiatry*, **2**, 750–6.

Coid, J. W. (1992) An effective syndrome in psychopaths with borderline personality disorder? *British Journal of Psychiatry* **162**, 641–50.

Cooper, J. L., Morrison, T. L. and Bigman, O. L. (1988) Bulimia and borderline personality disorder. *International Journal of Eating Disorders*, **7**, 43–9.

Copeman, J. P. and Zwanenberg, T. D. (1988) Practice receptionists; poorly trained and taken for granted? *Journal of the Royal College of General Practitioners*, **38**, 14–16.

Corney, R. H., Strathdee, G., Higgs, R., King, M., Williams, P., Sharp, D. and Pelosi, A. J. (1988) Managing the difficult patient: practical suggestions from a study day. *Journal of the Royal College of General Practitioners*, **38**, 349–52.

Cousins, N. (1982) Denial: are sharper definitions needed? *Journal of the American Medical Association*, **248**, 210–12.

Douglas, C. J. and Druss, R. G. (1987) Denial of illness; a reappraisal. *General Hospital Psychiatry*, **9**, 53–7.

Druss, R. G. and Douglas, C. J. (1988) Adaptive responses to illness and disability: healthy denial. *General Hospital Psychiatry*, **10**, 163–8.

Durkin, H. E. (1983) Some contributions of general systems theory to psychoanalytic group psychotherapy. In *The evolution of group analysis*, ed. M. Pines, pp. 76–97. London: Routledge and Kegan Paul.

Escobar, J. I., Burnam, M. A. and Karno, M. (1987) Somatization in the community. *Archives of General Psychiatry*, **44**, 713–18.

Fisher, G. C., Mitchell, I. and Murdoch, D. (1993) Munchausen's syndrome by proxy: the question of psychiatric illness in a child. *British Journal of Psychiatry*, **162**, 701–3.

Freeling, P. and Harris, C. M. (1984) *The doctor–patient relationship*, 3rd edn. Edinburgh, London: Churchill Livingstone.

Freidson, E. (1970) *The profession of medicine*. New York: Dodd Mead and Co.

Freud, S. (1910) *The future prospects of psycho-analytic therapy*, standard edn, Vol. XI, pp. 144–5. London: Hogarth Press.

Freud, S. (1912) *The dynamics of transference. General works*, Vol. *VIII*, London: Hogarth Press.

Friedman, H. (1969) Some problems of inpatient management with borderline patients. *American Journal of Psychiatry*, **124**, 299–304.

Frost, R. O., Morgenthau, J. E. and Riessman, C. K. (1986) Somatic response to stress, physical symptoms and health service use. *Behaviour Therapy and Research*, **24**, 569–76.

Gartner, A., Marcus, R., Halmi, K. and Loranger, A. W. (1989) *American Journal of Psychiatry*, **146**(12), 1585–91.

Gerrard, T. J. and Riddell, J. D. (1988) Difficult patients: black holes and secrets. *British Medical Journal*, **297**, 530–2.

Gerstley, L., McLellan, T., Alterman, A., Woody, G. E., Luborsky, L. and Prout, M. (1989) Ability to form an alliance with the therapist: a possible marker for prognosis in patients with anti-social personality disorder. *American Journal of Psychiatry*, **146**, 508–12.

Gillespie, R. D. (1929) *Hypochondria*. London: Kegan Paul.

GMC (General Medical Council: Education Committee) (1980) *Recommendations on basic medical education*. London: GMC.

GMC (General Medical Council: Education Committee) (1987) *Recommendations on the training of specialists*. London: GMC.

Graff, H. and Mallin, R. (1967) The syndrome of the wrist cutter. *American Journal of Psychiatry*, **124**, 36–42.

Green, S., Goldberg, R., Goldstein, D. and Leibenluft, E. (1988) *Limit setting in clinical practice*. Washington, DC: American Psychiatric Press.

Greer, S., Morris, T. and Pettingale, K. W. (1979) Psychological response to breast cancer: effect on outcome. *Lancet*, **2**, 785–7.

Grove, W. M. and Tellegen, A. (1991) Problems in the classification of personality disorders. *Journal of Personality Disorder*, **5**, 31–41.

Groves, J. E. (1978) Taking care of the hateful patient. *New England Journal of Medicine*. **298**, 883–5.

Hackett, T. P. (1969) Which patients turn you off? It's worth analyzing. *Medicine and Economics*, **46**(15), 94–99.

Hackett, T. P. and Cassem, N. H. (1974) Development of a quantitative rating scale to assess denial. *Journal of Psychosomatic Research*, **18**, 93–100.

Hackett, T. P., Cassem, N. H. and Wishnie, H. A. (1968) The coronary-care unit: an appraisal of its psychological hazards. *New England Journal of Medicine*, **279**, 1365–70.

Havers, L. (1968) Some difficulties in giving schizophrenic and borderline patients medication. *Psychiatry*, **31**, 44–50.

Havik, O. E. and Maeleund, J. G. (1980) Dimensions of verbal denial in myocardial infarction: correlates to three denial scales. *Scandinavian Journal of Psychology*, 27, 326–33.

Herman, J. L., Perry, J. C. and van der Kolk, B. A. (1989). Childhood trauma in borderline personality disorder. *American Journal of Psychiatry*, **146**, 490–5.

Heron, J. (1975) *Six categories of intervention analysis*. Guildford: University of Surrey.

Herzlich, C. (1975). *Health and illness*. London: Academic Press.

Horder, J. and Moore, G. T. (1990) The consultation and outcome. *British Journal of General Practice*, **40**, 442–3.

Jarvis, R. G. (1987) The 'tired person' syndrome. Understanding the pathologic factors in these 'problem' patients. *Postgraduate Medicine*, **81**(8), 321–4.

Kahana, R. and Bibring, G. L. (1965) Personality types in medical management. In *Psychiatry and medical practice in a general hospital*, ed. N. E. Zinberg, pp. 108–23. New York: International Universities Press.

Katon, W. (1984) Passion disorder and somatization: a review of 55 cases. *American Journal of Medicine*, **77**, 101–6.

Katon, W., Kleinman, A. and Rosen, G. (1982) Depression and somatization, a review. Part I. *American Journal of Medicine*, **72**, 127–35.

Kendell, R. E. (1972) A new look at hysteria. *Medicine*, **30**, 1780–3.

Kenyon, F. E. (1964) Hypochondriasis: a clinical study. *British Journal of Psychiatry*, **110**, 478–88.

Kernberg, O. (1975) *Borderline conditions and pathological narcissism*. New York: Jason Aronson.

Kessler, L. G., Cleary, P. D. and Burke, J. D. (1985) Psychiatric disorders in primary care. *Archives of General Psychiatry*, **42**, 583–7.

Kilpatrick, R. (1993) Rationale behind the General Medical Council's proposed new procedure for the assessment of doctor's performance. *British Journal of General Practice*, **42**, 2–3.

Kirmayer, L. J. (1984) Culture, affect and somatization. *Transcultural Psychiatric Research Review*, **21**, 159–88.

Kobasa, S. C. (1982) The hardy personality: toward a social psychology of stress and health. In *Social psychology of health and illness*, ed. J. Sules and G. Sanders. Hillsdale, NJ: Lawrence Erlbaum Associates.

Kuch, J. H., Schuman, S. S. and Curry, H. B. (1977) The problem patient and the problem doctor or do quacks make crocks? *Journal of Family Practice*, **5**, 647–53.

Langs, R. J. (1978) *The listening process*. New York: Aronson.

Levin, A. P. and Hyler, S. E. (1986) DSM-III personality diagnosis in bulimia. *Comprehensive Psychiatry*, **27**, 47–53.

Lewis, C. E. and Bucholz, K. K. (1991) Alcoholism, antisocial behaviour and family history. *British Journal of Addiction*, **86**, 177–94.

Lewis, G. and Appleby, L (1988) Personality disorder: the patients psychiatrists dislike. *British Journal of Psychiatry*, **153**, 44–9.

Lipowski, Z. J. (1988) Somatization: the concept and its clinical application. *American Journal of Psychiatry*, **145**, 1358–68.

Lipsitt, D. R. (1970) Medical and psychological characteristics of 'crocks'. *Psychiatry in Medicine*, **1**, 15–25.

Loeber, R. (1990) Development and risk factors of juvenile anti-social behaviour and delinquency. *Clinical Psychology Review*, **10**, 1–41.

Mace, C. J. (1992) Hysterical conversion. I. A history. *British Journal of Psychiatry*, **161**, 369–77.

Macleod, C., Mathews, A. and Tata, P. (1986) Attentional bias in emotional disorders. *Journal of Abnormal Psychology*, **95**, 15–20.

Main, T. F. (1957) The ailment. *British Journal of Medical Psychology*, **30**, 129–45.

Main, M., Kaplan, N. and Cassidy, J. (1985) Security in infancy, childhood and adulthood: a move to the level of representation. *Growing Points in Attachment Theory and Research in Child Development*, **50**, 66–106.

Martin, P. A. (1975) The obnoxious patient; tactics and techniques in psychoanalytic therapy. *Countertransference*, ed. P. L. Giovachin, pp. 196–204. New York: Jason Aronson.

McFarland, G. H., Freeborn, D. K. and Mullooly, J. P. (1985) Utilization patterns among long-term enrollees in a prepaid group practice health maintenance organisation. *Medical Care*, **23**, 1221–33.

McGaghie, W. C. and Whitenack, D. C. (1982) A scale for measurement of the problem patient labeling process. *Journal of Nervous and Mental Disease*, **170**, 598–604.

Meadow, R. (1977) Munchausen's syndrome by proxy – the hinterland of child abuse. *Lancet*, **ii**, 343–5.

Mechanic, D. (1962) The concept of illness behaviour. *Journal of Chronic Diseases*, **15**, 189–94.

Mechanic, D. (1970) Practice orientations among general medical practitioners in England and Wales. *Medical Care*, **VIII**(1), 15–25.

Menzies-Lyth, E. (1970). *The functioning of social systems as a defence against anxiety. A report on a study of the nursing service of a general hospital.* London: Tavistock.

Miller, L. J. (1989) Inpatient management of borderline personality disorder: a review and update. *Journal of Personality Disorders*, **3**(2), 122–34.

Nemiah, J. C. and Sifneos, F. G. (1970) Affect and fantasy in patients with psychosomatic disorders. In *Modern trends in psychosomatic medicine*, vol. 2, ed. O. W. Hill, pp. 26–34. London: Butterworths.

Norton, K. R. W., McGauley, G., Wilson, J. and Menzies, D. (1992) Health care services in the market place: early effects on caring relationships. *Therapeutic Communities*, **13**(4), 243–52.

Noyes, R., Reich, J. and Clancy, J. (1986). Reduction in hypochondriasis with treatment of panic disorder. *British Journal of Psychiatry*, **149**, 631–5.

Obholzer, A. (1989) Management of psychic reality. In *Contributions to social and political science*, pp. 119–28. Washington, DC: A. K. Rice Institute.

O'Dowd, T. C. (1988) Five years of heartsink patients in general practice. *British Medical Journal*, **297**, 528–30.

Paris, J. and Frank, H. (1989) Perceptions of parental bonding in borderline patients. *American Journal of Psychiatry*, **11**, 1498–9.

Parker, G., Abeshouse, B. and Morey, B. (1984) Depression in general practice. *Medical Journal of Australia*, **141**, 154–8.

Parkes, J. J. (1975) Psycho-social transitions: comparisons between reactions to loss of a limb and loss of a spouse. *British Journal of Psychiatry*, **127**, 204–10.

Parsons, T. (1951). *The social system.* New York: Free Press.

Pendleton, D. (1983) Doctor–patient communication: a review. In *Doctor–patient communication*, ed. D. Pendleton and J. Hasler, pp. 5–53. London: Academic Press.

Perry, J. C. and Klerman, G. L. (1980) Clinical features of borderline personality disorder. *American Journal of Psychiatry*, **142**, 15–21.

Perry, J. C., Lavori, P. W. and Hoke, L. (1987) Markove model for predicting levels of psychiatric service usage in borderline and anti-social personality disorders and bipolar type II affective disorder. *Psychiatric Research*, **21**, 215–32.

Pietroni, P. (1976) Non-verbal communication in the general practice survey. In *Language and communication in general practice*, ed. B. Tanner, pp. 162–79. London: Hodder and Stoughton.

Pilowsky, I. (1969). *Abnormal illness behaviour. British Journal of Medical Psychology*, **42**, 347–51.

Pope, H. G., Frankenburg, F. R., Hudson, J. I., Jonas, J. M. and Yurgelun-Todd, D. (1987) Is bulimia associated with borderline personality disorder? A controlled study. *Journal of Clinical Psychiatry*, **48**, 181–4.

Prestidge, B. R. and Lake, C. R. (1987) Prevalence and recognition of depression among primary care outpatients. *Journal of Family Practice*, **25**, 67–72.

Pringle, M., Bilkhu, J., Dorman, M. and Head, S. (1991) *Managing change in primary care.* Oxford: Radcliffe Medical Press.

Raczek, S. W. (1992) Childhood abuse and personality disorders. *Journal of Personality Disorders*, **6**, 109–116.

Reich, J., Yates, W. and Nduagaba, M. (1989) Prevalence of DSM-III personality disorders in the community. *Social Psychiatry and Psychiatric Epidemiology*, **24**, 12–16.

Robinson, D. (1971) *The process of beoming ill.* London: Routledge.

Roche, A. M., Guray, C. and Saunders, J. B. (1991) General practitioners' experiences of patients with drug and alcohol problems. *British Journal of Addiction*, **86**, 263–75.

Roukeema, R. W. (1976) The problem patient in your waiting room. *Journal of the Medical Society of New Jersey*, **73**, 985–8.

Royal College of General Practitioners (1972) *The future general practitioner: learning and teaching.* London: British Medical Journal.

Russell, D. E. H. (1983) The incidence and prevalence of intrafamilial and extra familial sexual abuse of female children. *Child Abuse and Neglect*, 7, 133–46.

Samuel, O. (1990) Towards a curriculum for general practice. *Occasional Paper*, **44**. London: Royal College of General Practitioners.

Savage, R. and Armstrong, D. (1990) Effect of a general practitioner's consulting style on patients' satisfaction: a controlled study. *British Medical Journal*, **301**, 968–70.

Schrire, S. (1986) Frequent attenders – a review. *Family Practitioner*, **3**, 272–5.

Schuller, A. B. (1977) About the problem patient. *Journal of Family Practice*, **4**, 653–4.

Schurman, R. A., Kramer, P. D. and Mitchell, J. B. (1985) The hidden mental health network. *Archives of General Psychiatry*, **42**, 89–94.

Shelp, E. E. and Perl, M. (1985) Denial in clinical medicine: a re-examination of the concept and its significance. *Archives of Internal Medicine*, **145**, 697–9.

Slater, E. (1965) The diagnosis of 'hysteria'. *British Medical Journal*, i, 1395–9.

Slavney, P. R. and Teitelbaum, M. L. (1985) Patients with medically unexplained symptoms: DSM-III diagnoses and demographic characteristics. *General Hospital Psychiatry*, **7**, 25–35.

Smith, R. J. and Steindler, M. S. (1983) The impact of difficult patients upon treaters: consequences and remedies. *Bulletin of the Menninger Clinic*, **47**, 107–16.

Stockwell, F. (1984) *The unpopular patient.* London: Groom Helm.

Strauss, D. H., Spitzer, R. L. and Muskin, P. R. (1990) Maladaptive denial of physical illness: a propoal for DSM-IV. *American Journal of Psychiatry*, **147**, 1168–72.

Szasz, T. A. and Hollender, M. H. (1956) A contribution to the philosophy of medicine. *Archives of Internal Medicine*, **97**, 585–92.

Turner, R. H. (1962) Role taking: process versus conformity. In *Human behaviour and social processes*, ed. A. M. Rose, pp. 20–40. Boston: Houghton Mifflin.

Tyrer, P. (1988) *Personality disorders: diagnosis, management and treatment.* London, Wright.

Tyrer, P. (1991) Neuroses and personality disorders. In *Concepts of mental disorder: a continuing debate*, ed. A. Kerry and H. McClelland, pp. 112–28. London: Gaskell.

Vaillant, G. E. (1971) Theoretical hierarchy of adaptive ego mechanisms. *Archives of General Psychiatry*, **24**, 107–18.

Vaillant, G. E. (1992) The historical origins of Sigmund Freud's concept of the mechanisms of defense. *International Review of Psycho-analysis*, **19**, Part 1.

Varsamis, J. and Adamson, J. D. (1976) Somatic symptoms of schizophrenia. *Canadian Psychiatric Association Journal*, **21**, 1–6.

von Bertalanffy, L. (ed.) (1973). *General systems theory. Foundations, developments, applications.* New York: George Braziller.

von Mering, O. and Earley, L. W. (1966) The diagnosis of problem patients. *Human Organization*, **25**, 20–3.

Wallen, J., Pincus, H. A., Goldman, H. H. *et al.* (1987) Psychiatric consultations in short term general hospitals. *Archives of General Psychiatry*, **44**, 163–8.

Weisman, A. D. (1972) *On dying and denying: a psychiatric study of terminality.* New York: Behavioural Publications.

Whitenack, D. D. and McGaghie, W. C. (1984) Towards an empirical description of problem patients. *Family Medicine*, **16**, 13–16.

WHO (World Health Organization) (1978) *Mental disorders: glossary and guide to their classification in accordance with the ninth revision of the International Classification of Diseases.* Geneva: WHO.

WHO (World Health Organization) (1992) *ICD-10 classification of mental and behavioural disorders. Clinical descriptions and diagnostic guidelines.* Geneva: WHO.

Widom, C. S. (1991) A tail on an untold tale: response to biological and genetic contributors to violence – Widom's untold tale. *Psychological Bulletin*, **109**, 130–2.

Wilson, A. (1991) Consultation length in general practice: a review. *British Journal of General Practice*, **41**, 119–22.

Wilson, D. R., Widmer, R. B. and Cadoret, R. J. (1982) Somatic symptoms: a major feature of depression in a family practice. *Journal of Affective Disorders*, **5**, 199–207.

Zimmerman, M. and Coryell, W. (1989) DSM-III personality disorder diagnoses in a non-patient sample: demographic correlates and comorbidity. *Archives of General Psychiatry*, **46**, 682–9.

Index

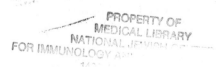